Understanding Breast Cancer

by Peter A. Dervan, M.D.

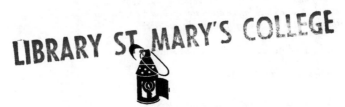
McFarland & Company, Inc., Publishers
Jefferson, North Carolina, and London

Library of Congress Cataloguing-in-Publication Data

Dervan, Peter A., 1945–
    Understanding breast cancer / by Peter A. Dervan.
        p.   cm.
    Includes index.
    ISBN 0-7864-1004-3 (softcover : 50# alkaline paper) ∞
    1. Breast—Cancer—Popular works.   I. Title.
    RC280.B8 D425   2001
    616.99'449—dc21   00-54808

British Library cataloguing data are available

Manufactured in the United States of America

Cover image: ©2000 Artville

McFarland & Company, Inc., Publishers
  Box 611, Jefferson, North Carolina 28640
    www.mcfarlandpub.com

Contents

List of Illustrations

Introduction

My first awareness of breast cancer came when I was a child, in the early 1950s. My grandmother died from it; she was in her 80s. At that time, cancer, like tuberculosis, was almost unmentionable. It seemed as if there was some shame attached to having cancer. It wasn't mentioned much in our house and as best I can remember it made little impact on me.

My next contact with this terrible disease came when I was a medical student, in the 1960s. First we learned about the pathology of cancer, and I remember being fascinated by this. All diseases were fascinating then, as we learned about them for the first time.

I do not recall being upset by cancer until I began my clinical work. Then it hit me. I was appalled by the number of patients we saw. Because we studied in a university hospital, we had a large number of referred patients. They often had advanced disease with little hope for the future. There was only one treatment then: mastectomy, and often this was a radical mastectomy (a mutilating operation).

Over the years, my interest in breast cancer has grown, not only from a professional viewpoint but also on a personal level. I have seen breast cancer strike my own family, my friends, my neighbors and my colleagues' wives.

As a surgical pathologist, I see breast cancer almost on a daily basis, and my professional interest has extended into our own research laboratory. Most of the research in my department relates to the molecular abnormalities in breast cancer.

Today, patients with advanced breast cancer do not fare much better than in my student days, despite many new treatments. However, major advances have been made in our understanding of how cancer grows and in the early detection and treatment of early and small cancers. Mammography detects the tiniest breast cancers before the patient or doctor

1

can feel them. Radical mastectomy is a procedure of the past and most patients are suitable for, and benefit from, breast-conserving surgery. Major advances in radiation therapy prevent recurrence after surgery. For some patients with more advanced disease chemotherapy is beneficial.

Most would agree that these advances have been only modest for the effort put into 30 years of intense research. However, during the past 30 years biomedical scientists have given us amazing new insights and an in-depth understanding of the genetic abnormalities in breast and other cancers. Our hope is that these new insights will lead to better treatments. Many believe that the information derived from the Human Genome Project and more genetic research will ultimately lead to a new era of gene therapy. They might be right.

Even if they are, however, these new treatments are decades away from finding their way into routine clinical practice. Even better than new treatments would be prevention. We are no nearer to finding the cause of breast cancer than were doctors 50 years ago. If we could find the cause, then we might have a chance of preventing the disease. That would be real progress.

I hope readers will find this small book useful and informative and that it will give them a cohesive overview of the many confusing topics they come across in newspapers and various media presentations. I have tried to keep the medical jargon to a minimum and have provided a glossary at the end of the book. The later chapters should be easy to understand and follow if the reader has read the early chapters first. I would advise readers to start at the beginning. I have tried to put the chapters in a logical order.

The many web addresses mentioned have a wealth of information not available in the best libraries in the best medical schools. However, readers should be aware that the Internet has its fair share of quacks offering unrealistic hope and sometimes dangerous advice. Try to stay with reputable sites—usually those hosted by government agencies, medical schools, and breast organizations.

The Scourge of Breast Cancer and the Scope of the Problem

There are three types of lies: lies, damn lies, and statistics.
—*Benjamin Disraeli (1804–1881)*

Breast cancer statistics are frightening and confusing, and there are many ways to present them. Look at the numbers here and see how they compare with any preconceived ideas you might have.

• Every twelve minutes, an American woman dies from breast cancer, and an additional four new patients are told they have this disease.

• In 1999, breast cancer struck approximately 176,000 American women and killed 43,000. Compare these to the fatalities in the Vietnam War from 1967 to 1975—there were 65,000 casualties.

• Breast cancer ranks just behind lung cancer as the leading cause of cancer deaths in women of all ages, and it is the leading cause of cancer deaths in women age 35–54 and the second leading cause of cancer deaths for women age 55–74 (Source: National Cancer Institute).

• Twenty-two percent of women with breast cancer are under the age of 50.

• Female deaths from breast cancer in the USA each year (approximately) in different age groups: all ages, 43,500; 75 and up, 13,800; 55–74, 19,900; 35–54, 9,200; 15–34, 600.

Studies carried out by the National Cancer Institute's Surveillance, Epidemiology and End Results (SEER) Program and mortality data from the National Center for Health Statistics (NCHS)[1-5] permit regular and consistent monitoring of cancer statistics and are an excellent source of information.

Statistics such as those above leave most people with little sense for the real or absolute risk to themselves. If you are on the high side of 40, chances are you know a family member, a friend, a relative, or a neighbor who has breast cancer. Cancer societies and the media tell us that 1 in 10 U.S. females, or 1 in 9, or even 1 in 8 get breast cancer. In the United Kingdom, the figure is 1 in 12. These figures, while accurate, are somewhat misleading.

Let's look at the statistics a little differently, by posing a question. Suppose you are a healthy female with no symptoms. What are the chances you will get breast cancer during the next ten years? A number of cancer registries have calculated the risks. As a woman enters her 30s, she has a 1 in 250 chance of getting breast cancer during the next ten years. As she enters her 40s, the risk over the next ten years is 1 in 75. During any ten-year period the risk never exceeds 1 in 35. Risk estimates depend on population statistics, and these vary slightly from country to country, from state to state, and on the techniques and methods used to gather them. The techniques used by biostatisticians are complicated, and not at all intuitive. The estimated risks (close approximation) at differing ages are shown in Table 1.1. Prior year statistics can be viewed in detail at the American Cancer Society web site (http://www.cancer.org/statistics). Because it takes a year or longer to collect and analyze data, "current" statistics always refer to events at least one year old (and often older).

What are the chances of getting cancer during the next year, if you are a woman, and age 30? Very slight, about 1 in 5,900. What about if you are 70? About 1 in 330.

Do men get breast cancer? Yes, most definitely; however, far less frequently than women. One percent of breast cancers occur in men and with the same devastating effects. In 1998, 1,300 American men got breast

Table 1.1	
Risk (females) of developing breast cancer during the next ten years	
If your age is now	Your chance of getting breast cancer during the next ten years is:
30	1 in 250
40	1 in 75
50	1 in 45
60	1 in 40
70	1 in 35

cancer, and 400 died (Source: National Cancer Institute). This book is about breast cancer in women; male breast cancer will not be discussed.

The public seems unaware that in the context of all diseases, the risk of death from breast cancer is relatively small. The average lady in the doctor's office, as she inhales her filtered cigarette, seems oblivious of the fact that (a) lung cancer kills more women than breast cancer (see figures 1.1 and 1.2), (b) 70 percent of patients treated for breast cancer survive ten years or longer, whereas lung cancer is curable in only about five percent of cases, and (c) lung cancer is largely preventable.

Even more deadly than all forms of cancer is cardiovascular disease (heart attacks and strokes). Yet, the public does not see these diseases with the same terror as cancer.[6] A mathematical model looking at a typical group of women adds some perspective to the figures.

The Ontario Cancer Registry, in 1995, looked at what was likely to happen to a group of 1,000 newborn females in the years to come. Eighty-five years later, 434 will still be alive. Along the way, 17 will die before the age 40 but none from breast cancer. This represents a typical but hypothetical group of 1,000 females. In practice, we know that when we study a population of millions, rather than 1,000, there will be some breast cancer deaths in this group. Getting back to the typical 1,000; during the next 20 years, nine will die from breast cancer (these are now women in their 40s and 50s), and during the next 20 years another 18 will die from breast cancer (women in their 60s and 70s). By the age of 85, breast cancer will have struck 99 women, and it will have killed 33. During the same time 203 women will have died from cardiovascular disease.[7,8] Of course, these figures do not take into account new discoveries and new therapies, which will undoubtedly improve survival during the next 85 years.

Most risks are expressed as relative risks. For the individual patient, absolute risk as it relates to herself is more important. It is possible to calculate the absolute risk from the relative risk, but few doctors know how to do this. There is a program available to download from a web site hosted by Vanderbilt University that allows them to do the calculations.

Leaving aside the mathematics of mortality, breast cancer has another devastating dimension. It lays heavy psychological, social, and financial burdens on victim, family, and society.[9-13] Once it strikes an individual, population statistics become somewhat irrelevant for the woman.

For the victim and her family there is a terrible uncertainty—the uncertainty of what will happen during treatment, what will happen when treatment is over, and what will happen in the long term. If the woman is the breadwinner, how will her disease affect her earnings? How will it

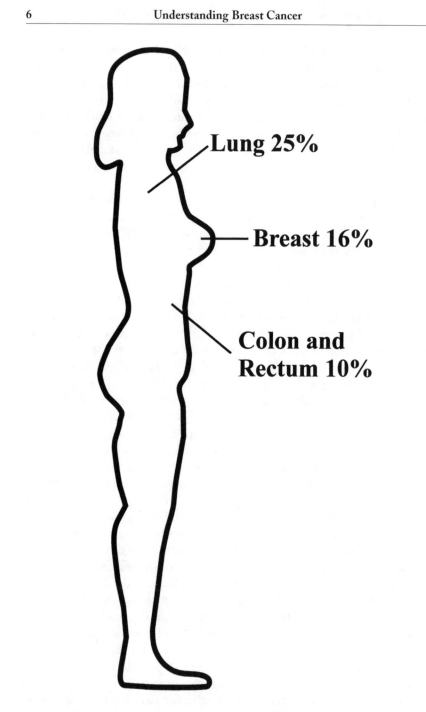

Figure 1.1   Cancer Deaths in Females

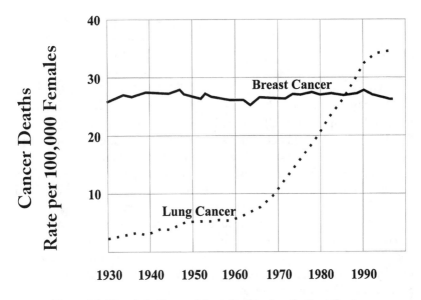

Figure 1.2 Trends in Cancer Mortality During the Last Century

affect her children? How will it affect her sexual and other relationships with her husband or partner? How will she cope with the stress of the disease and the therapy? If she has small children, who will look after them while she is ill? The people at Oncolink devote a large segment of their excellent web site to the psychosocial issues of breast cancer. They also provide book reviews devoted to these issues. (Further details on web sites are given in chapter 10.)

Ironically, some cancer patients acknowledge that their illness has brought a new meaning to their lives. It helps them psychologically. It helps them make profound decisions about their lives, decisions they had avoided for years or decades. Some women find inspiration and the time to do what they have secretly longed to do. Some write books, compose poetry, or become painters. Many find a new life helping others as voluntary workers.

The financial hardship on families is considerable but not accurately quantifiable.[14] The woman with cancer will have to take time off work, often for long periods. Her spouse may also miss time at work. Bank loans and insurance may be more difficult to get.

Breast cancer places a heavy burden on society and governments in terms of financial cost and research funding. The United States spends over $100 billion on cancer treatment each year. Loss of work costs $12 billion. Cancer screening, including mammography, Pap smears, colorectal examinations, and tests for prostate cancer, costs more than $4 billion. These figures are already out of date, and the cost of cancer care, like that of other diseases, is rocketing. New treatments and the ever-increasing cost of health care add to the financial burden on the state.

Are things getting better? Possibly. The American Cancer Society (ACS), National Cancer Institute (NCI), and Centers for Disease Control and Prevention (CDC) reported that cancer incidence and death rates for all cancers declined between 1990 and 1995, reversing a 20–year trend of increasing cancer cases and deaths in the United States.

Since 1991, the figures have continued to improve. While the incidence rates for breast cancer continue to rise, death rates have declined. The reduction in breast cancer mortality continued into the late 1990s, and is likely to continue into the 2000s. However, new analysis shows that recent improvements apply mostly to white women.[15,16] These changes may reflect (a) early diagnosis of preinvasive and small invasive carcinomas by mammography and (b) use of chemotherapy for early-stage disease. In the U.S., the improvement is seen mostly in white women who tend to have breast cancer diagnosed at an earlier (curable) stage. This in turn reflects the greater use of mammography by white women. In other Western countries, where mammography has been practiced for many years (such as Sweden), the declining mortality mirrors the trend in the U.S.[17]

Breast cancer vies with other major killers for research funds. In 1996, the NIH (National Institutes of Health) received $11.9 billion. They spent $0.38 billion on breast cancer research. In contrast, they spent $1.4 billion on AIDS (Acquired Immune Deficiency Syndrome) research. The benefits achieved by AIDS research far outweigh those achieved in cancer. In the past, AIDS was a death sentence. As a result of this research, many, if not most, AIDS patients can look forward to a cure. However, the fundamental problems in cancer are far more complex, and most experts admit that even if the same money were put into cancer research, it would be unlikely to achieve the same stunning results so quickly. We know what causes AIDS; it is HIV (the human immunodeficiency virus). We have a very poor understanding of what causes breast cancer. Knowing the enemy makes the likelihood of winning the war greater. Funding for research takes into consideration variables other than the incidence of disease, such as the likelihood of success.[18]

In summary, breast cancer is a major cause of morbidity and mortality; detection and treatment are improving; but we have a long, long way to go before we can eradicate this plague.

2

What Causes Breast Cancer?

Early this century, scientists discovered that something in mouse milk caused breast cancer in their offspring.[1,2] They thought they had discovered the cause of breast cancer in humans also. It was not to be.

For well over half a century the greatest scientific minds have struggled with the question, "What causes breast cancer?" During this time we sent men to the moon and robots to Mars. We developed amazing computer and telecommunications technology—witness the miracle of the Internet and the World Wide Web. We found the cause of tuberculosis, smallpox, and numerous other infectious diseases and conquered them. We are on the threshold of eradicating AIDS. We also learned to cure a small number of important cancers, such as Hodgkin's disease, childhood leukemia and testicular cancer. The war on cancer continues.[3,4] Yet, it is true to say that we are no closer today than we were 50 years ago to finding the cause of most breast cancers. Until we find the cause, it is unlikely that we will find a good cure, and it is inconceivable that we will be able to prevent it.

Although we have not yet identified the cause we have learned a great deal about its biology, especially during the past 25 years. Scientists have discovered the mechanisms of cell growth and aberrant cell behavior. They have discovered the biochemical machinery responsible for the behavior of normal cells, and they have identified the molecular mistakes that change a normal cell into a malignant one. If we consider the possible causes of breast cancer, we can conclude that: (1) the cause lies within ourselves, i.e., it is in our genes, or (2) the cause lies outside our bodies, i.e., it is in the environment. A third and more likely possibility is that it is some combination of both.

We know that some forms of cancer are inherited. These affect the intestine, kidney, thyroid gland, and eye. In fact, hereditary (genetic) cancers can arise in many different tissues, including the breast. Hereditary

9

breast cancers account for ten percent of all breast cancers. We know which genes are responsible for many of these and we know which molecules within these genes are damaged by the mutations we inherit from our parents. Furthermore, we can identify the mutations in a patient's and her relative's blood. Some researchers claim they can identify these mutations in cells scraped gently from the lining of the mouth, thus eliminating even the necessity for a blood test. These genetic abnormalities and hereditary breast cancers are discussed later in chapter 6.

Genetic abnormalities are complex. Genes control how our cells react to various noxious agents, including carcinogens. The biology becomes complicated when we realize that genes control other genes. A mutated gene anywhere in a tangle of DNA might be the trigger to start cells on their neoplastic journey.

Often the clue to the cause of disease comes from epidemiological studies. Epidemiologists are medical doctors and scientists trained in the use of biostatistics, and they spend much of their lives trying to find links between diseases and their possible causes. How do they do this? One popular way is by asking patients and normal people (those without the disease) to answer a detailed questionnaire. The questionnaire is worded skillfully to extract relevant information about what they eat and drink, where they work, or have worked, aspects of their family history such as the number of sisters or brothers they have, and whether any of them have had a similar illness. After various computer programs have examined the answers, the epidemiologists look for associations between the answers and the disease under investigation. They quantify, statistically, each association, in the hope that one or a few links stand out as more important than all the others. They give each association a "risk ratio." A risk ratio of 1 indicates that there is no difference between the diseased group and a carefully matched group of normal individuals. A risk ratio of 2 indicates twice the risk of the normal population. A risk ratio of 10 indicates that there is a strong link; they have 10 times the chance of normal individuals. Then the epidemiologists must look for a plausible explanation.

Suppose you are looking for the cause of infected toenails, and you are startled to find an association (with a risk ratio of 2) between cigarette smoking and sore toes. Perhaps the headlines say, "Today researchers found a link between cigarette smoking and infected toenails." You scratch your head and correctly conclude that this is probably nonsense. The association just doesn't appear to make sense. You look for other possible reasons to explain the statistics. You are likely to end up concluding that tight-fitting shoes are also linked and perhaps the groups of patients with the tight-fitting shoes are also heavy smokers. However, if you forgot to include a question relating to shoes, you might end up with a new hypothesis on the cause of infected toenails. In real life, unless you ask the correct questions you will end up with strange answers and possibly startling conclusions. To be taken seriously, statistical associations should also make biological sense.

After examining the results, epidemiologists may decide that a certain link is worth investigating further and repeat the study with certain modifications and refinements to get more accurate information. When you read a report that says people exposed to X, Y or Z are twice as likely to get cancer (risk ratio 2) than the normal unexposed population, you can usually ignore it. This apparent degree of risk could be real (but small). More likely, the result can be explained by bias or some confounding variable in the questionnaire. Unless you see a risk ratio of 4 or more you can conclude that the experts are not likely to take that threat seriously. Epidemiologists understand the limitations of their studies, and readily admit that theirs is an imperfect science.[5]

In contrast, journalists and those in the media desperately seeking a story often publish sensational headlines that bear no resemblance to reality. Perhaps their scare mongering is done in innocence or through lack of understanding. I doubt it. They need to sell news. How often have you heard something like this: "Yesterday, scientists at ABC medical center reported that they have found a link between XYZ and cancer." Such newspaper headlines are confusing to the public. As they read through the article they come across such words as "link," "association," "risk factors," and "risk ratio." Rarely do they know how little significance these terms have. Even the term "significant association" is statistical jargon and rarely means significant in the way we commonly use the word.

The type of study where patients are questioned about their lifestyle, and responses are compared to those who do not have cancer, is called a case control study. This is the most common type of epidemiological study. It is also the easiest to carry out, and the cheapest. Case control studies are less reliable than cohort studies and clinical trials. Cohort studies enroll thousands of normal individuals, sometimes as many as 100,000. At the beginning of the study these individuals have no evidence of the disease. They are questioned in depth concerning their exposure to as many risk factors as possible. During the years that follow, and at specific time intervals, researchers track their progress. Some develop cancer, some don't. The epidemiologists and biostatisticians then look for the links. For the past 30 years they have not come up with anything useful relating to the cause of breast cancer.

Theories regarding estrogen have been around since I was a medical student, back in the 1960s, and long before that. In fact, the estrogen theory has been around since the beginning of the century. Even before then there were clues. Observations made in 1713 by Ramazzini and in 1842 by Rigoni-Stern called attention to the fact that the incidence of breast cancer in nuns was much greater that in married women.[6] Epidemiologists work slowly.

Examples of cancer caused by something in the environment include skin cancer caused by sun exposure, mesothelioma caused by asbestos, and lung cancer caused by cigarette smoke. Although cigarette smoke causes approximately 90 percent of lung cancers, not everyone who smokes gets cancer. Some individuals are more susceptible than others to the inhaled carcinogens. Some individuals have a built-in defense mechanism that others lack. This defense is not an all-or-none phenomenon, but appears to be dose-related. Some individuals can absorb insults from the environment without significant tissue damage. Changes in our tissues and cells are often reversible, up to a point. Cells adapt to stress and injury. The lining of the lung can take a hammering from cigarettes for many years, with little visible damage. Cellular damage is subtle, cumulative, and often reversible. When an individual stops smoking, if he or she does so before the injury reaches a critical point, the lung lining reverts to normal. Stop smoking and your risk of getting lung cancer rapidly recedes. Cigarettes also cause crippling emphysema, and unfortunately, the damage is permanent. In other situations, a single insult, such as a blast of radiation, is oncogenic (cancer causing).

Although we cannot change our genes, we can readily change much of our environment. We can stop smoking, and we can legislate for the proper disposal of toxic waste products. The problem with breast cancer is that we do not know what causes the 90 percent of tumors that are not hereditary. If we could identify the environmental culprits, chances are we could prevent breast cancer. The logic of this last statement seems obvious. Nevertheless, we ignore the overwhelming evidence relating to cigarettes, and continue to poison ourselves. In 1997, 150,000 Americans died from lung cancer, almost all related to tobacco smoke.

• There are now 1.1 billion smokers in the world; this will rise to 1.5 billion by 2020 (Source: World Health Organization).

• There were 3 million smoking-related deaths per year in 1990; this will rise to 8 million by 2020 (representing 12 percent of all deaths) (Source: Harvard School of Public Health).

• Tobacco companies sell 5 trillion cigarettes annually.[7]

Although we do not know the cause or causes, epidemiological analyses of risk factors give us some clues. Cancer epidemiologists try to find statistical links between cancer and possible causes. They analyze as much data as possible, from as many different sources as possible, and hope to hit on some fact that ties in closely with disease. It is a bit like putting a jigsaw puzzle together. A little bit of information here and a little bit of information there gradually adds up to a whole picture. However, it is not as simple as that. A better analogy might be to try and build one picture from 100 or 1,000 different jigsaw puzzles all jumbled together in the same box. Even if the epidemiologists come up with the correct answer and find a plausible link, that is only the starting point. Nevertheless, it would be a crucial beginning. By dissecting the minute details of the association, scientists would then hope to find the ultimate culprit or culprits. This might be a virus, a chemical, or something totally different. It might be many different things.

For example, the association between mesothelioma and the shipbuilding industry led to the identification of the cause and subsequent prevention of this rare cancer. Malignant mesothelioma is a cancer of the outer lining of the lung. Epidemiologists found an unusually high incidence of mesothelioma in shipbuilders, a link with a specific occupation. Eventually, they found out that inhaled asbestos particles caused these tumors.

Asbestos mining began in 1878. Although doctors reported occasional cases of lung cancer in asbestos workers during the first half of the 20th century, the link between mesothelioma and asbestos did not become apparent until 1964.[8,9] Shipbuilders used asbestos in abundance. It was difficult to explain how some of their family members who did not work in the shipyards also got mesothelioma. Some sleuthing solved the puzzle. Workers in the shipbuilding yards brought asbestos fibers home in their clothes, and these fibers contaminated the air their families inhaled.

The link to mesothelioma and also to lung cancer led to a great reduction in the use of asbestos, and to improved health and safety regulations. Almost every country now restricts the use of asbestos. As a consequence, the incidence and mortality rates for mesothelioma have dropped dramatically.

In the mesothelioma example, epidemiologists identified patient's age, male sex, and occupation as risk factors. Middle-aged or older men with a long history of working in the shipyards were most affected. A confounding fact was that sometimes it appeared to occur also in patients who had very little exposure. As it turns out, many patients with mesothelioma had worked for only a short time with asbestos. Once asbestos is inhaled it remains embedded in the lungs for the rest of one's life. Like cigarettes, asbestos causes cancer in some people and not in others. Unlike tobacco, asbestos in small doses is carcinogenic.

We now know that many factors cause cancer. Scientists believe that our genetic makeup, in combination with external carcinogens, determine whether or not we are singled out. Not only the type of carcinogen, but also its dose is important. Matters are complicated by the fact that sometimes two or more environmental agents (cofactors) act in harmony to produce an additive effect. In other words, cigarette smoking in an asbestos worker has a much greater cancer-producing effect than in someone who is not exposed to asbestos. Cigarette-puffing asbestos workers have a much higher incidence of lung cancer than cigarette smokers not exposed to asbestos. And, cancer-smoking asbestos workers get lung cancer at a much younger age: cigarettes and asbestos are co-carcinogens. Some cancers may require more than two causative factors. Foods and vitamins, exercise, or 101 other variables that no one has yet thought about may also influence the risk for, or protect against, breast cancer. Such a complicated list of genetic and environmental interactions reminds one of the mathematical theory of chaos—apparently random events often have definite patterns if only we could understand them[10,11]; if only we could link the bits and pieces together we might find the cause. The principal suspects appear in Figure 2.1.

Risk Factors for Breast Cancer

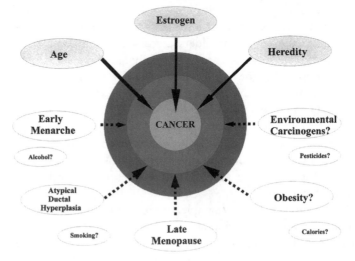

Figure 2.1. Age, prolonged estrogen exposure and heredity factors have the strongest links with breast cancer. There are many other statistical links, some of which are shown here—the smaller the size of the word, the weaker the link.

Estrogen

Breast cancer has many known risk factors (Table 2.1). Most known associations have a common link, namely, the hormone estrogen. Ovaries are estrogen factories, and between the ages of 14 and 45 they work at full production. Sometimes they continue to work in later life. Estrogen receptors sit on the outer surface of breast epithelial cells. They capture estrogen from the bloodstream and guide the hormone into the cell. Estrogen, along with many other stimulants, controls breast growth. Many risk factors point to a situation where there is heightened or prolonged exposure to estrogen.

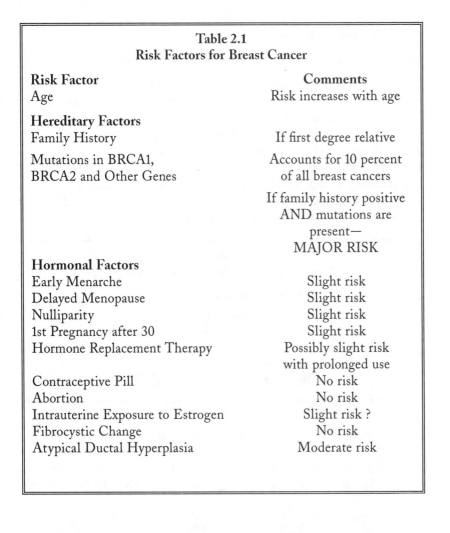

Table 2.1
Risk Factors for Breast Cancer

Risk Factor	Comments
Age	Risk increases with age
Hereditary Factors	
Family History	If first degree relative
Mutations in BRCA1, BRCA2 and Other Genes	Accounts for 10 percent of all breast cancers
	If family history positive AND mutations are present— MAJOR RISK
Hormonal Factors	
Early Menarche	Slight risk
Delayed Menopause	Slight risk
Nulliparity	Slight risk
1st Pregnancy after 30	Slight risk
Hormone Replacement Therapy	Possibly slight risk with prolonged use
Contraceptive Pill	No risk
Abortion	No risk
Intrauterine Exposure to Estrogen	Slight risk ?
Fibrocystic Change	No risk
Atypical Ductal Hyperplasia	Moderate risk

Table 2.1 (cont.)
Risk Factors for Breast Cancer

Dietary Factors

High Fat (calorie) Intake	Slight risk
Obesity	Slight risk

Environmental Factors

Breast Surgery	No risk
Cigarette Smoking	No risk ?
Pesticides	No risk ?
Alcohol	Slight risk?
Ionizing Radiation	Slight risk
Electromagnetic Fields	No risk

Some conditions protect against cancer. These are shown in Table 2.2. These too are linked to estrogen, or more specifically, to a lack of it. Early menarche (age of onset of menstruation) or delayed menopause means a greater lifetime exposure to estrogen. Anything that increases this exposure appears to increase the risk. Removal of both ovaries (oophorectomy) before the age of 30 has a pronounced protective effect.[12] Doctors use the drug Tamoxifen to prevent recurrent breast cancer. This blocks the uptake of estrogen by estrogen receptors and so prevents the hormone from entering tumor cells; it stops their continued growth.

Table 2.2
Factors Protecting Against Breast Cancer

Oophorectomy (removal of ovaries)
Delayed Menarche
Pregnancy before 30
Tamoxifen
Exercise
Breast feeding ?

Since the contraceptive pill and hormone replacement therapy (HRT) use estrogen, these would seem like logical risk factors. The facts tell us otherwise. Progesterone in the contraceptive pill balances and protects against the action of estrogen. Many studies show that the pill does not significantly increase the risk for breast cancer. Clearly, even if there is some risk, it is tiny. After some British newspapers exaggerated and sensationalized one study, the U.K. Committee on Safety of Medicines sent an urgent message to all directors of public health. They asked them to inform general practitioners and family planning doctors that there was no reason for women to stop taking the pill despite newspaper reports. In June 1996, The Lancet documented the background to this story in an editorial entitled "Pill scares and public responsibility."[13] In essence, the newspaper needed a "scare" headline to compete with news of an IRA carbombing in Manchester and news about a Russian election. Furthermore, careful analysis of the story in question revealed no "scare" information.

The evidence regarding hormone replacement therapy (HRT) is less straightforward. In 1997, a study in The Lancet pooled the results of 51 studies from all over the world, involving 160,000 women. It found a small risk confined to women on HRT for more than five years.[14] For long-term HRT users, there were 12 extra cases of breast cancer by the age of 70. This was 12 more than would be expected statistically for every 1,000 women who started taking HRT at the age of 50 and continued to take it for 20 years. There is no way of knowing if this survey over- or underestimates the true risk. These results did not distinguish between women on pure estrogen and those on a combination of estrogen and progesterone or one of its derivatives. Another study claims that cancers associated with HRT have a lower pathological grade than most breast cancers and by implication have a better prognosis—see chapter 9 on prognosis.[15]

In the same year, The New England Journal of Medicine reported the results of an HRT study in 120,000 nurses.[16] The Nurses' Health Study began in 1976 and looked at mortality rates in women on HRT in comparison to those not on hormone treatment. They found a lower mortality rate in HRT users. The benefit was likely due to reduced heart disease, or more specifically, reduced coronary artery disease; estrogen protects the coronary arteries from atherosclerosis. This study also found that hormone replacement for fewer than ten years lessened the risk of breast cancer, but increased the risk if used for more than ten years.

The exact risk associated with HRT use is unknown. Nine million American menopausal women take estrogen in the form of hormone replacement therapy. Does this cause breast cancer? Again, the results from various studies are somewhat conflicting. It is possible that HRT users are at some risk. However, this risk is small, and appears to be confined to long term use (more than five, or possibly ten years).[17] Experts agree that advantages of using HRT, in terms of alleviating postmenopausal symptoms and in preventing osteoporosis, greatly outweigh its slight risk.[16,18,19]

During pregnancy, another hormone—progesterone—seeps into the breast and this modifies how the breast responds to estrogen. Pregnancy before the age of 30 appears to alter the breast's response to estrogen. Some experts think that breast feeding also protects.[20,21] Other evidence suggests that breast feeding neither protects nor puts women at risk.[22]

Proliferative breast disease (also known as fibrocystic disease), when it contains abnormal cells (cytological atypia), is a risk factor. Pathologists call this atypical ductal hyperplasia (ADH). They have also identified some other low risk factors, which are mostly variants of fibrocystic change.[23–25] Fibrocystic change is one of the most common causes of a breast lump and experts believe it is caused by an uneven response of breast tissue to estrogen. Most patients with fibrocystic change are not at increased risk for malignancy.

For a time in 1997, a hotly debated issue was whether abortion predisposes to breast cancer. Some studies suggest it does. The explanation offered for this association was that normally in early pregnancy the breast is exposed to large quantities of circulating estrogen. As pregnancy proceeds, progesterone replaces estrogen and this resets breast cells to a more stable lifestyle. With early abortion, the breast is primed with estrogen but does not have the soothing effect of progesterone. Or so the story goes. However, more recent evidence strongly suggests that there is no definite association with abortion, that it is not a risk factor, and that the original research was flawed.[26–28] Most sensible obstetricians now accept this. The entire field of cancer risk is rife with rumor and conflicting studies, some showing that one variable is an important risk factor and subsequent studies casting doubt or disproving the association.

A mother's use of certain estrogen hormones during pregnancy increases the risk of vaginal cancer in the unborn female.[29] There is also a suggestion that exposure to estrogen before birth may increase the risk for breast cancer later in adult life.[30–32] This risk, if it exists, is very small. The oral contraceptive pill contains estrogen, and millions of women, worldwide, take it daily. After numerous conflicting studies the consensus opinion is that the pill does not predispose to breast cancer.[13] Some researchers think that oral contraceptive pills may even have a protective effect against ovarian cancer in patients with mutated BRCA1 or BRCA2 genes, the genes responsible for hereditary breast cancer (see chapter 6).[33] The other major component of the pill is progesterone, and like its effect in pregnancy, it appears to be protective.

The more scientists research the possibility that pesticides cause breast cancer, the less evidence they find. Each new study seems to refute previous links. Newer studies often address deficiencies or omissions in previous studies. So it is with electromagnetic fields (EMFs). Electromagnetic fields surrounding high-tension cables and generators have been the subject of emotive debate and dozens of cancer studies. Most have focused on their link with childhood cancer and in particular leukemia. Some epidemiologists and numerous pressure groups have long suspected a link between EMFs and cancer. Despite some lingering doubts, the current consensus opinion from the experts is that EMFs do not cause childhood cancers, breast cancer, or any other form of cancer.

What about obesity and alcohol? Fat cells, like the ovaries, produce estrogen. Some studies suggest that eating too many calories increases the cancer risk, and that exercise reduces the risk.[34,35] Believers think that diet and exercise can prevent breast cancer. However, this view is not widely held. At least one major study found no evidence for the fat intake theory.[36]

If estrogen is the main suspect in the breast cancer story, how then you might ask, could alcohol, pesticides, or other external agents cause breast cancer? Many agents can damage cells, and it is quite possible that there may be different mechanisms in operation in different patients. Alcohol, and possibly other chemicals, may modify, enhance, or alter estrogen metabolism in a number of different ways, so that the final common pathway is mediated by estrogen. The body modifies some chemicals in such a way that they resemble estrogens and trick breast tissue into seeing them as natural estrogens. Such chemicals have been called pseudo-estrogens or xeno-estrogens.[37,38] Perhaps cigarette smoke takes a similar estrogen-modifying route. Whichever way we look, there is always a hint that estrogen is in some way responsible for breast cancer.

Did you know that cigarette smoking probably plays a significant role in the onset of cancers other than lung cancer? It contributes to cancer of the mouth, cancer of the larynx (the voice box), and possibly also to cancer of the esophagus, pancreas, bladder, and breast. Its relationship to breast cancer is a new finding and not proven.[39] Dr. Timothy Lash from the Boston School of Public Health added fuel to the cigarette controversy by suggesting that smoking, whether active or passive, may contribute to breast cancer. He found the risk especially in girls exposed to cigarette smoke before the age of 12.[40] Dr. Alfedo Morabia and his colleagues in Switzerland also found an increased risk in passive smokers. Like other chemicals, such as pesticides, cigarette smoke changes estrogen metabolism. Some scientists postulate that the rising incidence of breast cancer may be due to increased smoking. Most medical and scientific communities remain highly skeptical and unimpressed with the smoking hypothesis.

Other variables subjected to epidemiological studies that have no link with breast cancer include breast augmentation surgery,[41] silicone-containing implants,[42] and fibrocystic disease (unless it is associated with atypical ductal hyperplasia). High dose ionizing radiation such as one gets from radiotherapy (or after a nuclear disaster) causes cancer in many tissues, including the breast. This risk is very low and for most women it is irrelevant. However, for one particular group of cancer patients it is a tragic complication of a life-saving treatment given at an earlier age. Hodgkin's disease is a cancer of the lymph nodes. It often strikes in the late teens or early 20s, and frequently involves lymph nodes hidden in the chest. The good news about Hodgkin's disease is that chemotherapy, radiation therapy, or a combination of both can cure most patients. Unfortunately, some young women who received radiotherapy to the lymph nodes in the chest subsequently got breast cancer years later.[43,44] They also got coronary artery disease.[45] Radiotherapy does a wonderful job killing the Hodgkin's disease. It also damages other tissues included in the radiation fields. In the future, greater use of chemotherapy and better radiotherapy techniques should remove the risk of these cancers. Unfortunately, chemotherapy also has its downside. Apart from its side effects during treatment, it too carries a risk for the subsequent development of cancer in other tissues, in particular the bone marrow. After high dose chemotherapy, some patients get leukemia in later life.[46-48]

Researchers in the past tried to implicate breast-screening mammography as a risky procedure. The amount of radiation delivered by modern mammographic machines is tiny, and we now know that clinical mammography is not carcinogenic.

Despite the popular opinion that psychological stress is responsible for all medical ills, there is no convincing evidence that stress causes breast cancer,[49] or for that matter, any other cancer.

The role of nutrition in the causation and possible prevention of breast cancer is under investigation. The results will not be known for many years. It will be surprising if this study provides any startling new insights into its cause.[50]

If you are a woman at normal risk for breast cancer, can you do anything to prevent it? Unfortunately, you can do nothing that will guarantee that you will remain cancer-free for the rest of your life. Doctors, gurus, or books that tell you otherwise are being less than honest. However, you can play the odds by living a healthy lifestyle in the knowledge that statistically this will place you in a group less likely to succumb. A healthy lifestyle means moderation in calorie and alcohol intake, and regular exercise. Fortunately, as you will see in chapter 5, you can do something to detect and cure breast cancer at an early stage by enrolling in a breast-screening program.

How Cancer Begins, Grows, and Spreads

The Normal Cell

To understand the mechanics of a cancer cell it is necessary to understand how normal cells work. The human body contains many organs, essential for life, such as the heart, brain, kidneys, liver, and lungs. Other organs, such as the ovaries, uterus, and breasts, while not essential, nevertheless enhance life. Each organ contains important tissues, and tissues are composed of cells.

Beneath the skin of the female breast lies a relatively simple anatomic but highly complex physiological structure (Figures 3.1 and 3.2). Fat occupies much of the breast. The remainder and most important part consists of specialized glandular tissue surrounded and protected by an envelope of connective tissue. The connective tissue consists mostly of a protein scaffolding called collagen, and it is similar to connective tissue elsewhere in the body. The ratio of glandular tissue to fat in young breasts is high and as a woman ages this ratio decreases; in later life, breasts consist mostly of fat. This fat to glandular ratio has some relevance to the usefulness of mammography in detecting early breast cancers and to the raging controversy about the value of mammography in younger women. I will discuss this in more detail in chapter 5.

The important structures within the breast are glands and the channels that connect them. These channels are the ducts. Cancer arises from the lining of the ducts and glands. In pregnancy, glands produce milk. Like a bunch of grapes dangling from twigs and stems, glands are connected to the nipple by a branching network of ducts; these ducts carry milk to the nipple. Bunches of glands are called lobules. Glands and ducts

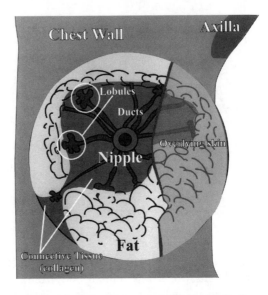

Figure 3.1. Breast with Outer Layer of Skin Partially Removed

have hollow centers, lined by epithelial cells.[1] These epithelial cells resemble those lining the stomach, intestine, lungs, or sweat glands in the skin. A layer of myoepithelial cells lies outside the epithelial cells. Myoepithelial cells have tiny contractile muscle filaments and they are responsible for propelling milk and secretions towards the nipple. The breast develops in the embryo from some unlikely structures; it grows from specialized sweat glands. During the miracle of embryogenesis, certain genes

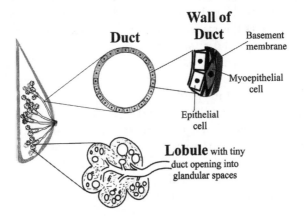

Figure 3.2. Glandular Tissue of Breast: Ducts and Lobules

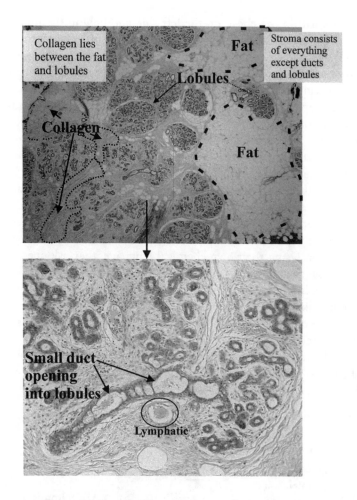

Figure 3.3 Breast—Normal Microscopic Appearance

program these sweat ducts to grow into breasts. A row of nipples appears in the young embryo, from the armpit to the groin. As the embryo grows, the extra nipples disappear. Rarely a little remnant persists into adult life; this is called an accessory nipple. Later, breasts grow and form under the influence of surging pubertal female hormones. A thin muscle wall surrounds ducts and glands. Between the epithelial cells and the muscle lies a sheet of basement membrane. This vital structure is critical in blocking cancer growth. As we will see later, it surrounds and walls off the early phase of breast cancer; it buys time for the patient, often years. Behind the breast lie the pectoral muscles, and behind these lie the ribs. The heart sits within the chest, on the left side and behind the inner part of the left breast. This relationship to the heart is of some importance, as we will see in a later chapter (see radiotherapy section in chapter 8). The armpit (axilla) contains important structures—the nerves and blood vessels supplying the arm, and lymph nodes.

Each epithelial cell functions like a busy little factory (Figure 3.4). In its center sits the control center—the nucleus. Here, genes send a constant flow of instructions to different components in the cell's main workplace, the cytoplasm. Cytoplasm, resembling a blob of jelly, surrounds the nucleus. A semipermeable membrane surrounds the cytoplasm and nucleus and keeps them separate from neighboring cells. Cells touch and stick lightly to their neighbors. Like tiles on a wall, these epithelial cells provide a smooth lining to the inner surface of the ducts and lobules. However, unlike tiles, they are alive. They grow and move, and they talk to one another. Using their own chemical language, they ask questions and send messages to their neighbors. They also respond to chemical changes in their environment and to stimuli from nutrients and hormones. Some of them make milk.

At the onset of puberty, the ovaries pour out estrogens. These immediately enter the bloodstream and make their way to the, as yet, tiny breasts. Here, estrogen locks onto receptors embedded in the outer wall of the breast cells and triggers the cells to grow, and grow, and grow. They continue to grow until they reach normal adult size. For the rest of the

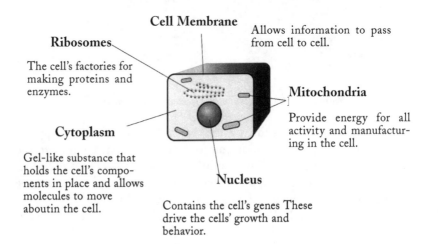

Cell Membrane
Allows information to pass from cell to cell.

Ribosomes
The cell's factories for making proteins and enzymes.

Mitochondria
Provide energy for all activity and manufacturing in the cell.

Cytoplasm
Gel-like substance that holds the cell's components in place and allows molecules to move about in the cell.

Nucleus
Contains the cell's genes These drive the cells' growth and behavior.

Figure 3.4. Epithelial Cell

woman's reproductive life her breasts respond to waves of estrogen. The second most important female hormone (also from the ovary) is progesterone and it acts in harmony with estrogen. Depending on whether it is early or late in the menstrual cycle, estrogen or progesterone will play the dominant role. Another hormone, prolactin, from the pituitary gland located at the base of the brain, is responsible for breast growth during pregnancy. Prolactin instructs breast cells to make milk.

Throughout a woman's reproductive life, from menarche to menopause, hormones ebb and flow. Each month of her menstrual cycle brings to her breasts a cyclical flood of estrogen and progesterone. In response, breast tissue swells and shrinks slightly. Many women feel their breasts uncomfortable or painful just before menstruation. Some women have discomfort beginning at the time of ovulation, two weeks before menstruation. Mostly it is fluid retention from the hormonal changes that causes the discomfort. The breast is far removed from the ovaries, which are deep in the pelvis. Yet, these almond-shaped little organs exert immense influence on everything a breast cell does, from age 12 until the menopause (and sometimes beyond that).

The Cancer Cell

A normal breast cell has many responsibilities. It must talk to its neighbors, grow in an organized, coherent fashion, respond to cyclical signals from its environment, and when the time is right make milk. Cells, in order to work properly, make proteins and other essential molecules. Genes provide blueprints for making these molecules. Whenever the need arises, genes instruct ribosomes, floating in the cell's cytoplasm, to make new proteins, such as enzymes. They tell the mitochondria, "We need to do some more work. Can you please speed up your energy supply?" Or, when cell metabolism slows down, when the brain falls asleep, it says, "Okay, take a break. We don't need so much oxygen for a few hours." All day and all night, 365 days a year, every cell in the body, all 300 billion of them, continuously check their immediate environment. They receive and respond to signals from cells located in distant organs.

Normal breast epithelial cells go about their daily duties quietly and without fuss. They live in harmony with their neighbors. When cancer strikes, a single cell turns delinquent and behaves badly. It no longer responds to the rules and needs of its community. At first, a single epithelial cell, lining one of the ducts, disregards instructions regulating growth and behavior. It becomes independent, and gradually it and its family and their offspring destroy the breast tissue. Biologists call this extended family a clone (Figure 3.5). Malignant tumors are monoclonal, i.e., they come from one (mono-) bad cell. Up to 1 billion cells live in a small malignant tumor, and these all come from a single cell and its descendants. In contrast, benign tumors consist of clones derived from numerous cells and their families; they are polyclonal. Cancer cells are dangerous because they can spread to other organs—lymph nodes, lungs, bones, and brain. They squat there, then grow and kill normal cells, and eventually the patient.

Although scientists have not found the cause of breast cancer, they now believe they understand most of the inner workings of the cancer cell. They view cancer progression as an infinite series of ministeps, with each evolutionary step furthering the tumor's progress.

For ease of study, they categorize carcinogenesis into three major events: initial preinvasive growth, invasion, and metastasis. However, each category contains many genetically controlled separate steps. For the past 30 years, biology and medical research laboratories world-wide have struggled to find out what exactly controls each of these steps.[2] Dedicated doctors and post-doctoral students work late into the night and give up their weekends in search of the answers. Pharmaceutical giants, along with the U.S. and most other governments, and charities large and small, have poured hundreds of billions of dollars into cancer research. Although not widely appreciated, they have had remarkable success.

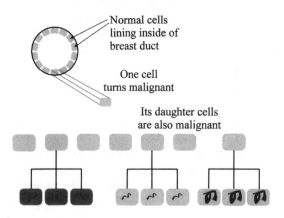

Normal cells
lining inside of
breast duct

One cell
turns malignant

Its daughter cells
are also malignant

Subsequent offspring (clones) are also malignant.
Some clones develop different malignant characteristics

Figure 3.5. Clones of Malignant Cells

The fruit of their research is a gigantic reservoir of information detailing the structure and function of the normal cell and all its components, and how these go wrong in cancer cells. Nevertheless, we still have enormous gaps in our knowledge. Critics complain that medicine has moved too slowly and that scientific information has not been translated into useful practice, namely cures. To some extent they are correct. When President Richard Nixon launched the war on cancer in 1971 with massive research resources, few understood how complex the normal cell was, or how much more complex the cancer cell was.

Within the nucleus of each cell, 23 chromosome pairs lie tangled like a ball of thread (Figure 3.6). Chromosomes consist of protein scaffolding, wrapped in a chemical known as deoxyribonucleic acid or DNA (Figure 3.7). DNA's single most remarkable characteristic is that it can reproduce itself, precisely. This substance is responsible for identical twins and cloned animals. It also lies at the heart of cancer. This wonder compound consists of a sugar molecule (deoxyribose), phosphate, and four chemicals called adenine, thymine, cytosine, and guanine, more commonly known as A, T, C, and G. These are entwined to form a structure like a

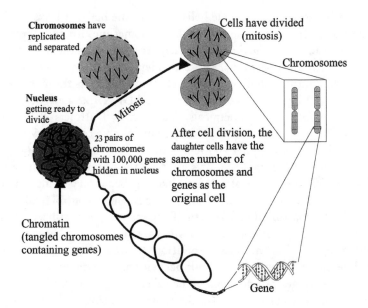

Figure 3.6. Chromosome and Gene Replication During Cell Division (Mitosis) Contains 23 pairs of chromosomes. During cell multiplication chromosomes replicate, and mirror copies go into the daughter cells (upper part of illustration). Genes reside in the chromosomes and identical genes are present in every cell.

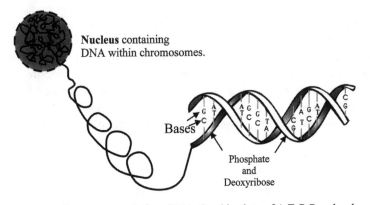

Nucleus containing
DNA within chromosomes.

Bases

Phosphate
and
Deoxyribose

All genes are made from DNA. Combinations of A T C G molecules
form the genetic code. This code writes messages which are
translated into proteins. Wrong codes allow the cell to grow uncontrolled.
Uncontrolled growth results in cancer.

Figure 3.7. DNA

spiral staircase; this is a double helix. Within the helix, A links to T, and
C links to G. In most tissues, at regular (or sometimes irregular) intervals,
cells divide and form daughter cells. Each time the parent divides it replaces
itself with two daughter cells. These are identical to each other and to the
parent cell. During cell division, each chromosome splits through the center of its DNA helix. Each strand of unzipped DNA, like a magnet, attracts
opposite complementary chemicals; A attracts T, T attracts A, C attracts
G, and G attracts C. A complicated group of tools called enzymes control this delicate unzipping and rebonding. They glue the bits and pieces
together so that the final products are two mirror images of the original
DNA. Individual chunks of DNA sit like tiny beads on a string, and each
bead has a different function.[3] These are genes. Genes control fetal growth;
in fact, they control all cell growth. They instruct cells to become bone,
brain, or breast. This specialized process whereby cells become one or
another organ is known as differentiation. As we will see in a later chapter, differentiation influences tumor behavior and treatment.

Genes trigger cell division. Some cells, such as neurons in the brain,
never divide after birth. Others, like those producing the oxygen-carrying red blood cells, live such a hectic lifestyle that they must divide every
day. Others enjoy a more leisurely existence and reproduce once a week
or once a month. Still others don't bother to divide until some outside
signal encourages them to replicate.

Like a computer network, signals flow to and from cells scattered throughout the body. Computer instructions move a humble computer mouse, or a robot on Mars. They also command the pixels on a screen to show a beautiful landscape or an intricate drawing. Computer language has only two numbers, "0" and "1." All computer data and instructions come from some unique combination of the digits 0 and 1. In contrast, DNA has four letters, A, T, G and C. By using groups of any three letters, and by varying the number of groups, DNA has an infinite vocabulary. And it writes the instructions for life.

A wrong computer digit can have disastrous consequences. A wrong code might tell a missile to destroy a target—but the wrong target. So too a DNA error may have devastating consequences for a cell and its owner. A wrong amino acid code, resulting in an abnormally shaped red blood cell, condemns its owner to live and die with sickle-cell anemia (amino acids are the building blocks for proteins). A different mistake results in hemophilia. Inherited genetic damage prevents hemophiliacs from making an essential blood-clotting protein. In the past, this condemned young boys to repeated hemorrhages into joints and other tissues, to lives of painful destructive arthritis, and eventually to death. Modern medicine ensures that these boys grow into men and live normal lives. Like diabetics they need life-long injections, not of insulin, but the purified blood-clotting factor, factor VIII.

Different sets of A, T, C, and G make different amino acids. Different amino acids combine to form different proteins, and these send different signals and messages. The entire process is complex, fine-tuned, and self-regulating. A wrong word, an extra word, or a lost word in a sentence may radically alter its meaning. Compare "Mrs. Jones did not show up last night" with "Mrs. Jones did show up last night." Lose that three-letter combination "not" and you tell a lie about Mrs. Jones. Consider the significance of two lost letters in these sentences: "The biopsy showed no cancer" and "The biopsy showed cancer." Imagine the disastrous treatment that could follow such a typographic error. In the language of DNA and genes, mistakes and their messages can also have disastrous consequences—they give rise to cancer.

Among the unanswered questions 30 years ago were "what causes cancer?" and "How does it cause cancer?" Unfortunately, we have made little headway in answering the first question. However, unprecedented breakthroughs in molecular biology, and many clever new techniques, allow us to look in submicroscopic detail at the inner workings of the cell. In particular, these techniques allow us to examine genes and how they work. Already, scientists can remove and insert DNA into individual cells.

They can manipulate DNA and fuse it with other bits of DNA to clone new DNA. Dolly, the cloned sheep, highlighted the power of cloning. Cloning scientists are attempting to make human organs in the hope that they can replace damaged hearts, lungs, and livers. If they are successful, "spare part" cloning will provide an endless supply of organs, and the need for donor organs may disappear.[4] Medical and scientific optimists hope that these techniques will repair or replace damaged DNA and will eventually cure cancer. I will discuss recent advances in gene therapy in the final chapter.

DNA unzipping and zipping results in cell division and new cells. From time to time, minor degrees of slippage occur along the double helix. Specialized enzymes snip damaged DNA fragments and replace them with newer molecules. They also repair mismatched AT and CG pairs. Throughout life, the cell feels many stresses and it copes very well most of the time. What happens if the DNA damage goes too far and the fix-it enzymes can no longer repair the damage? Another set of genes becomes active. These are "suicide" genes and they quickly compel the cell to self-destruct. Scientists call this process of self-destruction apoptosis.[5-10] After apoptosis is complete, macrophages, the scavenger cells of the immune system, move in, remove the dead cell, and bury it in its reticulendothelial system. This system contains demolition cells known as macrophages, and lymphocytes (immune cells) in the lymph nodes, spleen, and in other tissues scattered throughout the body.

Apoptosis also occurs in healthy cells when they reach old age or when they need to renew themselves. The term apoptosis comes from the Greek "apoptos" meaning "to drop off." Just as old leaves drop from a tree, so too, old cells fall away from a normal organ. Apoptosis plays a major role in young developing tissue. In fact, it is one of the main mechanisms whereby fingers and toes and many organs form in the developing embryo. The apoptotic process chips away unwanted cells from primitive limbs as other embryonic genes sculpt perfect diminutive fingers and toes. Apoptosis is critical for cancer growth.

Fundamental information, emerging from 30 of years research, indicates that genes control every step and ministep. Different genes control cell division, tumor growth, invasion, and metastasis. To date, scientists have identified hundreds of damaged genes that influence and control cancer behavior. The following section will focus on just a few of the better-known genes and what they do.

There are four major categories of cancer controlling genes—oncogenes, tumor suppressor genes, apoptosis-controlling genes, and mismatch repair genes.[11] These control normal cell growth and only cause a problem when they are damaged or malfunction. Oncogenes and tumor suppressor genes are the cells' accelerators and brakes. They act in unison to drive a cell smoothly. Too much pressure on the accelerator genes drives the cell into uncontrolled growth. The same thing happens if the suppressor brakes are jammed. Heightened oncogene activity, or reduced tumor suppressor activity, ends with a cell speeding out of control. Mismatch repair genes scan and monitor DNA replication. When they detect a mistake they remove the damaged gene segment and replace it with new DNA.[12,13] Mutated repair genes don't work properly and allow accelerated growth.

One of the most common oncogenes activated in breast cancer is HER-2/neu (also known as c-erbB2). This gene makes a receptor protein on the outer surface of the cell membrane.[14] Like a magnet sticking out from the cell, it attracts and binds chemicals known as growth factors.[15] The receptor structure is such that only chemicals with the proper molecular shape can bind successfully—similar to how a key fits into a lock. The correct combination sends a message to the cell nucleus that activates another gene, and this accelerates cell growth. Overactive, uncontrolled HER-2/neu gene activity covers the cell surface with too many receptors, which in turn bind too many growth factors, which in turn feed the nucleus with signals to grow and multiply. This oncogene also improves the tumor cell's motility; it helps it to crawl away from its neighbors and move along the breast duct. As discussed in the chapter on treatment, a new drug, Herceptin, can inactivate the properties of HER-2/neu.[16] The mechanisms whereby other oncogenes activate breast epithelial cells often differ from each other. Sometimes the oncogenes produce more growth factors on the cell surface; sometimes they send signals that increase the activity of proteins or enzymes within the cell (Figure 3.8a).

The best-known tumor suppressor gene is the p53, and it lives on the short arm of chromosome 17. It functions as the "guardian" of the genome, by monitoring and protecting dozens of cell growth mechanisms.[17] Loss of normal p53 activity allows a dozen or more control mechanisms to break down. More than half of all cancers, including breast cancer, have damaged p53 genes.[18-24] Mostly, external agents cause p53 damage. Rarely, patients inherit p53 mutations and have a tendency to develop multiple cancers. These patients have the Li-Fraumeni syndrome.[25]

An army of enzymes and genes oversee and control cell growth, keeping a proper balance between cell loss and cell gain. Despite these protective safeguards, the DNA replicative and signaling systems are not fail-safe. From time to time, minor DNA mistakes slip by undetected. Often these have no serious consequences. However, some DNA errors

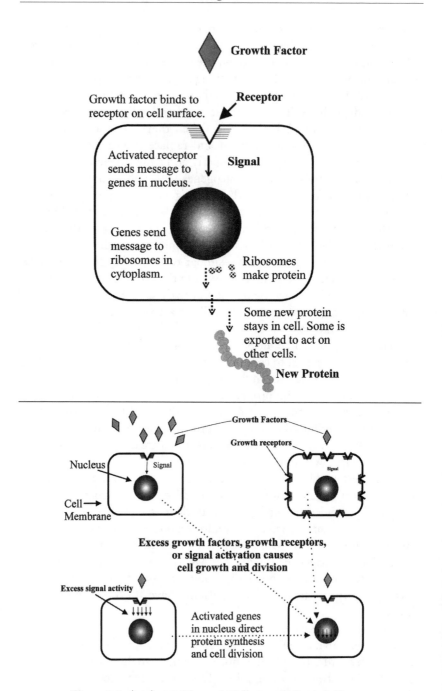

Figure 3.8a (top) *and Figure 3.8b* (bottom).*Growth Factors*

set up a cascade of miscoded signals that eventually convert the cell and its offspring into a malignant tumor. Carcinogenesis, in many respects, mimics accelerated evolution.[26] Each new mistake in the cascade confers some advantage on the new cell; otherwise, it is eliminated. The fittest survive. This cell no longer requires the same oxygen or nutrition as its neighbors. It grows bigger, stronger, and aggressive. Unrestricted by surrounding cells, it moves about more freely. Its offspring and their subsequent families become dangerous aggressors.

Normal tissues maintain their size by finely tuning the balance between cell accumulation and cell loss. If you examine a cross section of skin in a microscope, you will see that cells along the bottom layer of the epidermis are dividing, whereas those in the upper layer are dead and falling from the surface. We constantly shed the outermost layer of skin. The time from cell division to cell death is only ten days. In some skin disorders, such as psoriasis, cells grow more quickly than normal and die in about four days. Because of the rapid growth, cell accumulation exceeds cell loss—the result is a build-up of cells on the surface. This causes the white shiny scale so characteristic of psoriasis.

Tumors grow because cell accumulation exceeds cell loss (Figure 3.9). As mentioned above, apoptosis controls cell loss in normal tissue. The best-known apoptos-controlling gene is bcl 2.[27,28] This and a host of other genes (including p53) interact to induce programmed cell death; scientists like to call this cell suicide.[29-31] These cells are not killed by anything outside the cell. They self-destruct. Mutated, inactivated apoptotic genes contribute to tumor growth. They cannot make the tumor self-destruct as cells do in normal tissue.

Unlike normal cells, cancer cells can live forever. Perhaps not forever. Nevertheless, they can grow indefinitely in the laboratory. Put cancer cells into culture dishes, feed them regularly, and they will survive and grow strong, long after the patient is dead. HeLa tumor cells crawl around petri dishes in many cancer research centers and laboratories throughout the world. These cells came from Henrietta Lack. This 31-year-old Baltimore woman died from cervical cancer in 1951.

A recently discovered mechanism explains why cancer cells live longer than normal cells.[32-36] The tips of each chromosome, known as telomeres, contain unique DNA sequences that control cell aging. Every time a cell divides it loses a little telomeric DNA. As cells continue to divide they lose more and more telomeres and they age and stop dividing. The telomere is the cell's biological clock.[37] The enzyme telomerase prevents telomere shortening and is absent in normal adult cells. Guess what scientists found in cancer cells? They found telomerase, present and work-

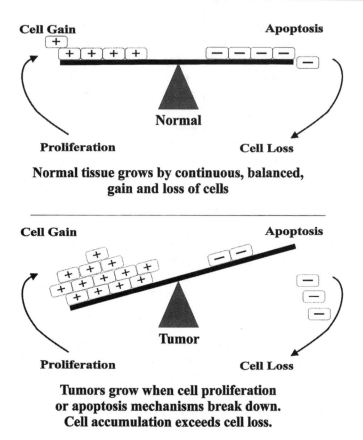

Figure 3.9. Tumor Growth

ing overtime.[38] Dividing cancer cells keep their telomeres intact; they remain young forever and achieve immortality (at least in a test tube). Clearly, many factors other than telomerase influence cell mortality. Early hopes that telomerase activation in tumor cells could be used as a target for treatment have not yet shown much promise.

Malignant changes evolve as a continuous process, beginning with a clonal overgrowth of the first abnormal cell. Early, only its internal molecular clock is abnormal. At this stage, a pathologist examining such a cell through the most powerful microscope on the planet would not detect any abnormality. Sometime later, perhaps in one or two years, the clonal offspring appear slightly abnormal. These cells are larger than their neighbors, and their nuclei look darker and have a coarser texture. At this stage, an experienced pathologist will recognize the abnormality. A biopsy report will use words such as cellular atypia, dysplasia, or more commonly, atypical ductal hyperplasia, to describe the cells. Even these rather late changes (from a molecular viewpoint) often do not progress to cancer. The body's defense mechanisms can remove some or all of the dysplastic cells. Often these abnormalities regress, or progress no further. However, if they continue to grow, at some stage they reach a critical point from where they cannot return. In time, dysplastic cells become malignant cells. This is carcinoma in situ. When tumor cells remain confined to the ducts, i.e., when they have not penetrated the basement membrane, the pathologist's report will say "ductal carcinoma in situ" (Figure 3.10). The patient may not appreciate it when she first hears this diagnosis, but, relatively speaking, ductal carcinoma in situ is good news. It means that she will be cured, and more often than not, without losing her breast.

Within the duct, carcinoma cells behave like European cuckoos, crowding out normal law-abiding epithelial cells. After a few years' residence in the confines of the hollow breast ducts, some cells grow restless and need more freedom. Uncontrolled growth, while important, is in some respects far less important than another deadly property. If a tumor grew indefinitely, but remained where it began, treatment would be easy. Local excision would be curative. Far more important than a tumor's longevity or its growth rate is its ability to invade and destroy normal tissue and then travel to distant organs.

If they wish to move outside their ducts, tumor cells must learn to do two things. They must learn to crawl and they must learn how to break through the basement membrane barrier. In the language of biomedicine this crawling is termed "cell motility." If you take a group of normal epithelial cells and place them in a petri dish, they will grow as a tightly molded, orderly, regimented colony. If you do the same experiment with malignant epithelial cells, they will soon take off in all directions, like wild uninhibited delinquents on open ground. They will move away from the main group, and movement is often random and unpredictable. Normal cells obey messages and instructions from their "motility" genes, and move in unison with the purpose of a swarm of ants or bees. Many genes (including HER-2/neu) contribute to abnormal motility.[39,40] These genes modify the cell's internal molecular skeleton and foot-like processes (pseudopodia) on the cell's outer wall. Cell adhesion molecules coat the outer surface of each cell and these molecules glue cells to their neighbors, neatly and tightly (Figure 3.11). Similar but sturdier Velcro-like hooks strengthen the bonds between cells, and anchor cells to the underlying basement membrane. These hooks are desmosomes.

In malignant cells, mutated genes fail to make adhesion molecules,

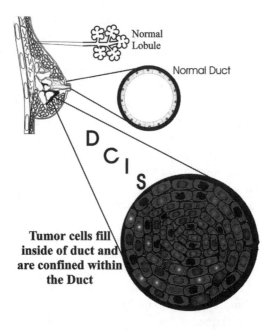

Figure 3.10. Ductal Carcinoma in Situ

or make bad molecules that do not function properly.[41-45] No longer constrained by a coat of zippers, cells begin to crawl in all directions. As they develop their motility skills, they move along the basement membrane.[46] In the meantime, a different set of mutated genes start up the enzyme factories that would normally be active only in inflammatory demolition cells and some immune cells. Such enzyme production is appropriate and desirable in inflammatory cells, whose role is to destroy bacterial invaders, but not in epithelial cells. When they are fighting bacteria, these enzymes are invaluable. The differentiation genes, mentioned earlier, ensure that such enzymes lie idle in normal breast epithelial cells. When activated and secreted by tumor cells these enzymes create havoc and play a critical role in helping cancer cells destroy the basement membrane.

A constant stream of mutations equips malignant cells with these new weapons—proteolytic destructive enzymes. Tumor cells then secrete these enzymes, and they dissolve the surrounding protective basement membrane. Punched-out holes and cracks appear in this membrane, and the more aggressive cells slither through into the connective tissue space that surrounds the ducts. They invade the stroma (Figure 3.12). They have now won a major battle. While they remain inside the ducts they cannot metastasize. However, once they penetrate the ductal basement membrane they can flee from the confines of the breast.

As the hole-punching gang moves along the breast duct, crawlers squeeze through tiny basement membrane gaps. Like an amoeba, cell after cell slithers from ducts into the surrounding stroma. Suddenly they find themselves in the wide open space of the breast stroma. This is not really wide open space but a jungle of connective tissue surrounded by fibers and gel. Most of the fibers are collagen, a tough mesh-like protein present in all tissues. Slowly, inexorably, tumor cells latch onto the collagen and other fibers in the stroma and they dissolve the surrounding gel.[47] Collagen has many functions, but in the breast it mostly acts as scaffolding to support and protect the epithelial-lined ducts and lobules. Other essential structures, like nerves, lymphatics, and blood vessels live entwined in the collagen meshwork.

Once the tumor breaks through the basement membrane, it is an invasive carcinoma and the patient's battle against cancer now enters a new and dangerous phase. Within the stroma lie exit channels and pathways to lymph nodes, lung, and liver, and to all other organs. To help them penetrate these exit vessels they demolish existing barriers by releasing more destructive enzymes.[48-50]

As they move through the stroma, they build their own new scaffolding, often in great abundance. This framework consists mostly of a different type of collagen, and this gives a firmness or hardness to the tumor. It is this hardness that allows a patient, nurse, or doctor to feel

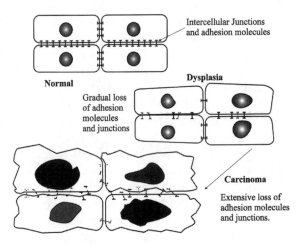

Figure 3.11. Cell Adhesion

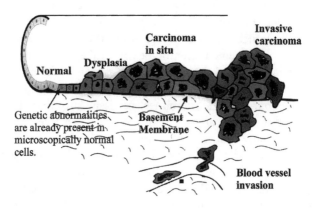

Figure 3.12. Progression from Normal to Invasive Cancer

and identify a tumor. This collagen also helps the cancer to bind firmly to surrounding tissues, such as skin or underlying muscle. If they can feel the tumor, doctors say "it is palpable." However, long before it becomes palpable it can often be detected by mammography. For this reason, screening programs use mammography to identify in situ and early invasive cancers.

Invasive tumor cells grow relentlessly and spread within the breast, usually slowly but sometimes rapidly. An invasive tumor the size of a pinhead (1-2 mm) already contains a few million tumor cells. As tumor cells continue to mutate, their evolutionary tricks allow them to invade lymphatics and tiny veins. Fragile thin-walled lymphatics provide less resistance to invaders than blood vessels, and so tumor cells usually infiltrate these first. Sometimes however, they invade blood vessels before or simultaneously with lymphatics. Once they gain access to lymphatics they are free to travel to lymph nodes in the armpit (the axilla), or behind the breast, within the chest. Vascular invasion gives them access to the cardiovascular system. Wherever blood travels (everywhere) cancer cells can now go.

When cancer has metastasized by the bloodstream, it has almost won the battle. But not quite. At every step of its progression, the body tries to stop and destroy the invader. Even after the tumor has metastasized, the body continues to do battle. After metastasizing, some tumor cells die, and some hibernate for months, years, or even decades.[51,52] Nevertheless, when breast cancer travels to tissues other than lymph nodes it is difficult to eradicate. Most patients with metastases to lungs, liver, bone, or brain will die from their disease. There are many exceptions. Chemotherapy, even if it fails to carry out its prime function—to kill all metastatic cells—sometimes forces tumor cells to become dormant. Sleeping tumor cells (if they remain asleep) may let the patient live a normal lifespan.

Just as dozens of genes working together control growth, so too a cascade of mutated genes direct basement membrane destruction, and lymphatic and vascular invasion. While thousands of scientists study the mysteries and secrets of cell growth, their colleagues in nearby laboratories focus their research on invasion. The cancer cell's most deadly characteristic is its ability to metastasize. Metastases kill. Apart from destructive enzymes and cell motility which are crucial for invasion, cancer cells need some additional properties to help them spread.

One of these is the ability to trick lymphatics into thinking that tumor cells are lymphocytes. Lymphocytes are immune cells that patrol the body and destroy foreign molecules. They live in lymph nodes. Lymph nodes lie hidden throughout the body. Those guarding the breast reside high up in the axilla (armpit). The last place tumor cells should seek refuge is in a lymph node. Nevertheless, this is where they usually go first. Normal lymphocytes carry, on their outer membrane, a receptor known as CD44.[53] This is its identity card. It allows the lymphocyte to slip in and out of the lymph node unchallenged. Tumor cells do not normally carry an identity card. However, they forge one. By changing their differentiation codes, they can make CD44, identical to the receptor on lymphocytes. This disguise allows them to travel into and around the axillary lymph nodes. Once inside, like the enemy in a Trojan horse, they begin to grow, proliferate and destroy the lymph node.

In recent years, researchers have pinpointed new blood vessel formation or neoangiogenesis (neo = new, angiogenesis = blood vessel formation) as a critical step in the metastatic process. Normal cells require oxygen and food. The oxygen we breathe binds tightly to hemoglobin in our circulating red blood cells. These cells visit every nook and cranny in every tissue and organ, and deliver life-supporting oxygen. They reach their destination by a meshwork of large, small, and tiny blood vessels (capillaries). These same capillaries carry food and essential nutrients such as vitamins, water, and minerals from the intestine. They also carry essential hormones. Cells lining the inside of blood vessels are called endothelial cells. A trillion endothelial cells line these blood vessels. They stretch over an area of 1,000 square meters, the estimated surface area of the body's vascular system. Normally, these are slow growing, stable cells. When stimulated they proliferate rapidly—as rapidly as bone marrow cells, if necessary—and they make new vessels. Tumors can grow to approximately 2 to 3 mm^3 without a blood supply. Tumors this size contain about

1 million tumor cells. Tumors larger than this need their own blood supply (Figure 3.13). By secreting a chemical growth factor called tumor angiogenesis factor (TAF), cancers trick surrounding normal tissue into supplying them with new blood vessels. Without its blood supply a tumor would suffocate and die. In its early stage of invasion, until it is about 2 mm, it can live off existing capillaries. However, as it outgrows its existing blood supply it must make its own new blood vessels.[54–56] In the near future, some treatments may target these blood vessels, the idea being to cut off the tumor's fuel supply.[57,58] Endothelial cells have unique molecules on their surface known as endoglin and endosialin. Scientists believe that these molecules are different from those on the endothelial cells of normal blood vessels. If so, they may become suitable targets for new therapies. Pharmacologists will try to make antibodies to these molecules and tag them with cytotoxic drugs or radioactive isotopes. They will then fire these "magic bullets" specifically at tumor endothelial cells, and at the same time avoid normal blood vessels and their lining cells. If they succeed in destroying endothelial cells, the tumor vessels will self-destruct and isolate the tumor from its essential oxygen and nutrients.

However, do not be surprised if they fail. Evolution is amazing, even within the microcosm of a tumor. Put an obstacle in front of a tumor and

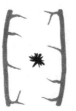

Small invasive tumor surrounded by normal blood vessels.

Invasive cancers larger than 2mm can make their own new blood supply. These blood vessels grow in response to chemicals secreted by the tumor cells.

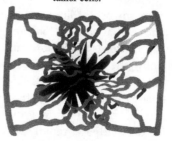

Figure 3.13. Tumor Angiogenesis

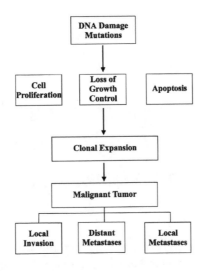

Figure 3.14. Carcinogenesis

gradually mutations in a few cells will often allow it to find the ways and means to overcome the problem. New mutations will allow a few cells to overcome the obstacle and begin growing again. Someone once said a tumor behaved "a bit like an automobile coming to a wall and then growing helicopter wings to get over it." Cutting off the tumor's blood supply sounds like a wonderful idea. It might work, if the vessels can be destroyed abruptly. Give the tumor cells time and they will find ways to overcome the reduced blood supply. Already we have clues that tumor cells might be able to survive oxygen deprivation. Many tumors need less oxygen than normal cells. It is possible that further mutations will allow them to survive total oxygen deprivation.

Apart from the genes controlling angiogenesis, it appears that many other aberrant genes contribute to metastases. Some have already been identified. The gene nm23 (nm stands for nonmetastatic) helps normal cells to differentiate and mature. Mutated nm23 is found in many metastatic cancers.[59,60] However, how it contributes to metastases is poorly understood.

Over the past few years, scientists have built genetic profiles of large numbers of cancers and compared slow growers to rapid growers, invaders to non-invaders, and metastasizers to non-metastasizers. Using this information they gradually hope to unravel the mechanisms of metastases. By understanding the precise mechanisms involved in tumor progression (cell growth, invasion and metastases), scientists believe they can design the best anticancer treatments. Figure 3.14 summarizes the main cellular events in cancer progression from a normal cell to distant metastases.

The Pathology of Breast Cancer: How It Looks Under the Microscope

Tumor terminology is often confusing and uses long and difficult words. The ending on the word usually gives a clue to the meaning. Words ending with "-oma" usually refer to tumor. Occasionally, -"oma" also refers to tumor-like lumps. For example, a granuloma is a tumor-like inflammatory lesion that one finds in some diseases, e.g., tuberculosis. If you come across a word that ends in "-itis," this means inflammation. Although not often used nowadays, mastitis means inflammation of the breast.[1,2]

These are the common conditions affecting the breast:

- fibroadenoma
- cysts
- fibrocystic disease (also called fibrocystic change)
- duct ectasia
- fat necrosis
- specific inflammations, such as breast abscess or tuberculosis (very rare)
- carcinoma of various types
- other benign and malignant tumors

Virtually any abnormality in the breast can produce a terrifying lump. The more common causes include cysts, fibrocystic disease, fat necrosis, fibroadenomas, and carcinomas. Other conditions causing a breast lump would fill a large textbook, but most of these are very rare. The likelihood of the lump being malignant is influenced somewhat by the patient's age. In young women, under the age of 40, most lumps are benign. In older women, a larger percentage is malignant.

Benign Breast Diseases

Fibroadenomas

Fibroadenomas affect all age groups. These harmless lumps are often as small as a pinhead and live unnoticed in normal breasts. The larger ones become pea- or grape-sized and produce a palpable lump, or reveal themselves in a mammogram. Uncommonly they reach the size of a golf ball.

Most fibroadenomas are so characteristic clinically that the doctor can often make a confident diagnosis just by examining the breast. Classically, the fibroadenoma measures 1 to 2 centimeters and is firm and well demarcated from the surrounding breast tissue (Figure 4.1). One important sign is that it moves freely. It is not bound down to nearby tissue and tends to slip away from the examining fingers. Some surgical textbooks refer to fibroadenoma as a "breast mouse," darting back and forth beneath the examining fingers. It also has a characteristic appearance on a mammogram where it produces a well-defined round or oval shadow with nice sharp margins. If there is the slightest doubt about the diagnosis or the slightest hint that it might be something worse, the doctor will advise biopsy or removal. Even if the clinical diagnosis seems straightforward, the patient usually will want to get rid of it for peace of mind. Old surgical textbooks often advised removal of fibroadenomas "as no lady should have lump in her breast." A surgeon can remove a fibroadenoma easily and leave no cosmetic damage apart from a tiny skin scar.

The macroscopic appearance is characteristic. A fibroadenoma consists of firm tissue surrounded by a very thin, often shiny, membrane; this is the connective tissue capsule that separates it from surrounding tissue. The capsule, as it were, holds everything in and allows the surgeon to pop out the fibroadenoma from normal breast tissue. Its appearance under the microscope gives it its name, being composed of fibrous tissue (fibro-) and benign glandular tissue (-adenoma). These two components are intermingled in different proportions. Pathologists sometimes subclassify fibroadenomas depending on the microscopic growth patterns. The subclassifications have no relevance for the patient. Some patients may have more than one fibroadenoma and occasionally these involve both breasts. They do not always appear at the same time. Some women will find new fibroadenomas a few years after the original one was removed. A diagnosis of fibroadenoma brings relief to the patient and her family; it is perfectly benign and not premalignant.

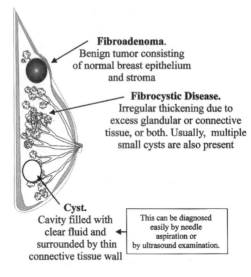

Fibroadenoma.
Benign tumor consisting
of normal breast epithelium
and stroma

Fibrocystic Disease.
Irregular thickening due to
excess glandular or connective
tissue, or both. Usually, multiple
small cysts are also present

Cyst.
Cavity filled with
clear fluid and
surrounded by thin
connective tissue wall

This can be diagnosed
easily by needle
aspiration or
by ultrasound examination.

Figure 4.1. Benign Breast Lumps

Cysts

A cyst is a dilated segment of duct filled with protein-rich fluid (Figure 4.1). Some physiological kink in the duct prevents normal drainage. As secretions from the epithelial cells accumulate they fill and expand the duct. Microscopically, normal duct epithelial cells line the cyst wall. If a cyst is large enough (usually greater than one centimeter) it can produce a lump. A surgeon examining such a lump will usually conclude that because it is well circumscribed it is benign. The main clinical differential diagnosis is fibroadenoma. Its appearance may not be as definitive as the fibroadenoma because smaller cysts at its edge can produce an imperfect margin as they merge with surrounding tissue. The surgeon confirms the diagnosis simply by inserting a needle and aspirating it. As clear fluid fills the syringe the cyst collapses, the lump disappears, and the diagnosis becomes instantly obvious. Usually, the patient needs no further treatment other than reassurance. Cloudy or blood-stained cyst fluid, or persistence of the lump after aspiration, raises the suspicion of malignancy in the surgeon's mind. Only a biopsy will now give the definitive diagnosis. Rarely, benign cysts and carcinoma can coexist. The size of the cyst can mask the presence of a small carcinoma. When the cyst is aspirated and it collapses the nearby carcinoma may become obvious. Ultrasound examination is also ideal for diagnosing cysts.

Fibrocystic disease

Despite its name, this is not a disease; up to 20 percent of female breasts, at autopsy, have it.[3,4] A more accurate term is fibrocystic change, and the changes are normal physiological changes. Gradually the term "change" is replacing the word "disease" in medical breast terminology. However, when these changes are exaggerated they produce a lump. Often the lump is obvious, or it may be so ill defined the patient says she can feel it even if the surgeon cannot. Although fibrocystic disease commonly affects women around the menopause, it occurs at any age.

Fibrocystic change has many microscopic faces. These include a combination of abundant glands interspersed between small cysts and dense fibrous tissue. The name of the process comes from the combination of fibrous tissue (fibro-) and cysts (-cystic). An older term placed more emphasis on the glandular proliferation and called it fibroadenosis. Older medical literature called it chronic mastitis or mammary dysplasia (not to be confused with the premalignant change, with the same name, described in chapter 3).

Macroscopically, fibrocystic change produces a vague "rubbery" thickening of few or many areas in the breast, accompanied by small and large cysts. The histologic appearance has a wide spectrum of changes. At one extreme, the changes are so subtle that it is difficult to distinguish it from normal breast. At the opposite extreme it closely mimics cancer. Most cases lie comfortably in between and produce characteristic readily identifiable microscopic changes. Some variations of fibrocystic change have their own names. These include sclerosing adenosis, blunt duct adenosis, and apocrine metaplasia. As its name suggests, sclerosing adenosis consists of abundant glandular proliferation and a prominent fibrous reaction. In the past (pre 1970s) before this variant of fibrocystic disease was widely recognized, sclerosing adenosis was sometimes misdiagnosed as cancer. Unfortunately, such a misdiagnosis led to unnecessary mastectomy.

Rarely, the cells lining the glands show such abnormal nuclei that their interpretation causes diagnostic problems. The dilemma for the pathologist is whether such changes represent early malignant change (ductal carcinoma in situ) and should be reported as such. The term used for this abnormality is atypical ductal hyperplasia (ADH). Such cases often call for a second opinion. When many pathologists examine the same tissue from such specimens they frequently disagree on a precise diagnosis, i.e., whether the change represents ADH or carcinoma in situ. In medical-statistical parlance, this condition has a high incidence of inter-observer variability. The real problem stems from the fact that there is a continuum of change from normal epithelium to ductal carcinoma in situ (DCIS) and the biopsy might have come from the edge of something more sinister. Atypical ductal hyperplasia represents dysplastic change that occasionally progresses to malignancy. However, in any particular case it is not known whether it will progress or not.

This microscopic confusion leaves the surgeon with two dilemmas. What will he tell the patient, and what further treatment is needed? Should he biopsy again, to ensure that there is no cancer adjacent to the atypical hyperplasia, or should he adopt a wait and watch policy? In practice, a combination of factors will dictate the next move—the extent and severity of the atypical hyperplasia, the clinical findings, the mammographic appearance, the age of the patient, and the patient's wishes. The type of biopsy in which the ADH was found will also influence the next move. If the biopsy was a needle biopsy (a small sample), then the chances of finding DCIS in a repeat open biopsy or excision are fairly high (up to 30 percent chance.[5] An open biopsy will almost always follow after a needle core shows ADH.

Strange as is may seem, if the ADH was found as an incidental finding buried in the middle of fibrocystic change, in an open biopsy, the chances of finding anything worse in a repeat excision are negligible. In this situation the surgeon and the patient will opt for continued observation and follow-up rather than another biopsy. In terms of risk, the presence of ADH in fibrocystic change in an excision specimen means that the patient has about four times the normal chance of having breast cancer sometime in the future. This risk involves both breasts, not just the breast and the area from which the ADH came. If ADH seems confusing to you, you have every right to be confused. So are the experts.

In the past, epidemiologists and biostatisticians argued about the risks for subsequent carcinoma in patients with a diagnosis of fibrocystic disease. It is obvious now that ordinary fibrocystic disease without ADH carries no significant risk. The increased risk is confined to patients with fibrocystic disease in combination with ADH, and possibly sclerosing adenosis.

Breast Cancer Classification

Pathologists classify breast cancer under two major headings, and a variety of subheadings (Figure 4.2). The major headings are in situ

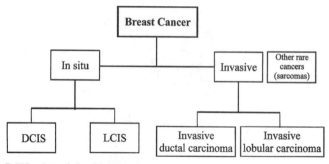

DCIS = Ductal Carcinoma in Situ
LCIS = Lobular Carcinoma in Situ

Figure 4.2. Classification of Breast Cancer

carcinoma and invasive carcinoma. The distinction is critical. In situ carcinomas cannot spread outside the breast—they have no metastatic potential—and complete removal is curative in almost every patient. In contrast, invasive cancer can metastasize widely and kill the patient.

In situ carcinomas are subclassified into lobular carcinoma in situ (LCIS) and ductal carcinoma in situ (DCIS). Even though neither metastasize, their distinction from each other is important as their risk for progression and their treatments differ radically.

Lobular carcinoma in situ is clinically and mammographically silent. It produces no symptoms and no signs, and makes itself known to the pathologist as an incidental finding on the microscope. As the pathologist scans back and forth across the abnormal "lump," a few breast lobules located in normal tissue attract the examining eyes. These are large (two or three times the size of a normal lobule) and they are filled and distended with small round cells that show little or no nuclear abnormalities (Figure 4.3). They are remarkably innocuous looking. Although the LCIS lobule is large, relative to the size of normal lobules, its absolute size is no more than a few millimeters. Nevertheless, in the past, LCIS has caused intense debate among pathologists and surgeons with ensuing extreme differences in treatment. Differing attitudes to LCIS resulted in radical recommendations, ranging from doing nothing to performing a bilateral mastectomy. The "do nothing" group has won out in the end. The current recommendation from almost all experts is that these patients should not have mastectomy but should have long-term careful observation, similar to that for any patient with increased risk.

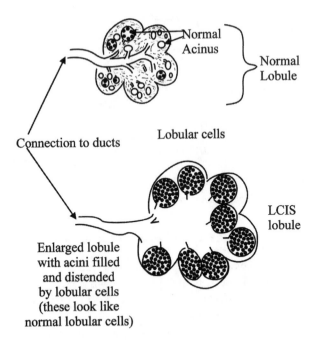

Normal
Acinus

Normal
Lobule

Connection to ducts

Lobular cells

LCIS
lobule

Enlarged lobule
with acini filled
and distended
by lobular cells
(these look like
normal lobular cells)

Figure 4.3. Lobular Carcinoma in Situ (LCIS)

When LCIS first came to the attention of pathologists in the 1940s, its significance was poorly understood. Epidemiologic data in the 1970s suggested that patients with LCIS had an exceptionally high risk of developing invasive carcinoma at a later date. So threatening was this perceived risk of subsequent cancer by some surgeons that one famous New York hospital promoted and performed bilateral prophylactic mastectomy. However, surgeons at another famous hospital felt so strongly about its lack of threat that they removed the word carcinoma from the term LCIS. They suggested that the term lobular carcinoma in situ should be named lobular neoplasia in situ.

LCIS is not immediately life threatening; it cannot metastasize, and progression to invasive cancer is not inevitable. In fact, most patients with LCIS never get invasive breast cancer. The true incidence of LCIS is unknown and varies from study to study.[6] We know that the risk for getting invasive cancer sometime in the future is about nine times normal.[7,8] Because it is multifocal and often bilateral, a subsequent carcinoma can affect any part of either breast.[9]

Under the microscope LCIS involving a few lobules resembles a coss section of a small bunch of grapes. Each grape represents a distended acinus. Imagine a grape, bulging with too many seeds but held in place by an intact outer layer of skin. In LCIS, each acinus is bulging with too many cells and these are contained by the basement membrane. The appearance of each cell does not deviate greatly from its benign counterpart in a normal acinus. Nevertheless, these cells have grown out of control.

We know that LCIS rarely progresses to invasive cancer. Nevertheless, for some women it indicates a significant risk for breast cancer sometime in future. What it tells us is often frustrating and annoying. It says, "The good news is this: I am not very likely to come back at all. However, rarely, I do return and then I am just as dangerous as any other cancer. Furthermore, there is nothing you can do, short of removing both breasts, to prevent me from doing so. If I return, you may find me just beside the original biopsy site. Then again, I'm just as likely to return in a different part of the breast, or even in the other breast." In the face of such a diagnosis there is little the surgeon can do other than advise the patient to have long-term follow-up. Hopefully, if an invasive cancer develops subsequently it can be detected and removed at an early stage. The surgeon will try to explain the facts as reassuringly as possible, so as not to induce a lifelong anxiety about a possible but unlikely recurrence sometime in the future. In exceptional circumstances, the pathologist might report LCIS involving a large number of lobules, rather than the usual few. If this happens, the surgeon may advise removal of some more breast tissue surrounding the biopsy site to make sure that it does not contain a small invasive cancer.

If LCIS recurs as an invasive cancer, intuitively we would expect this to be an invasive lobular carcinoma. However, sometimes it recurs as a different type of cancer—invasive ductal carcinoma. I will discuss this shortly. In essence, what LCIS tells us is that some unknown carcinogen is targeting the epithelial cells lining this woman's ducts and lobules. In some women, over the period of years one of these cells eventually loses its normal growth-regulating properties and becomes malignant. This may happen anywhere in either breast. For these reasons many experts suggest that LCIS should be regarded as a risk factor rather than a true carcinoma in situ. Carcinoma in situ would be expected to progress and become invasive eventually at its original site.

The important message regarding LCIS is that it does not metastasize, normally does not require any further surgery, does not require radiotherapy or chemotherapy, and rarely becomes invasive. In contrast to LCIS, in situ carcinoma involving the duct system, i.e., ductal carcinoma in situ (DCIS), is common and less controversial. It has the potential to progress in a "logical" fashion to invasive cancer and requires complete removal.

When pathologists review the total number of breast cancers they see each year, they find that about 15 percent of them are DCIS. Fifteen years ago that number was only five percent or less. Some of this increase is apparently due to a genuinely increased incidence of DCIS. However, the increase is mostly due to the widespread use of mammography, which detects early breast cancer.

Twenty, or even ten years ago, when pathologists found DCIS in a breast biopsy they reported it as DCIS, without attempting to subclassify it. Surgeons, when they got such a report, did a mastectomy. We now know that for most women mastectomy is unnecessary. Pathologists and surgeons also recognize that there are different forms of DCIS, with different levels of aggressiveness. These have some bearing on how the patient will be treated.

As its name implies, DCIS is cancer confined within the lumen of the breast ducts (Figure 3.10). It has a number of different growth patterns—giving rise to the terms comedocarcinoma, solid, cribriform and micropapillary variants of DCIS. Usually DCIS involves only the ducts in one segment of the breast (Figure 4.4). With such localized disease breast-conserving surgery is curative, and mastectomy is unnecessary. A small number of patients have extensive DCIS throughout the breast, and they need a simple mastectomy.

Sometimes the pathological distinction between DCIS and (benign) epithelial hyperplasia is difficult and requires an opinion from an expert

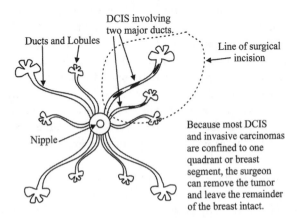

Figure 4.4. Breast-Conserving Surgery

with a large DCIS experience. Such experts are found in university medical centers caring for large numbers of patients with breast disease. They often also have a special academic interest in breast pathology, and many participate in breast cancer research programs. However, usually the pathological diagnosis is relatively straightforward. Pathologists grade DCIS depending on the degree of cell, or more specifically, nuclear abnormalities they view under the microscope.[10–13] There are a number of different classification systems, but essentially they all indicate whether the in situ cancer is high grade or low grade. High grade DCIS is more likely to recur, and after surgery the patient often receives radiotherapy to the breast to prevent such recurrence. Sometimes patients with low grade DCIS also receive radiotherapy, but its value in low grade DCIS is debatable.

Within the medical world, pathology is often regarded as the most "scientific." When the science is put to the test it sometimes fails. Like all branches of medicine good pathology practice consists of a mixture of art and science. Every so often, pathologists come across a particularly difficult case and have to decide whether a biopsy shows DCIS or an extreme form of hyperplasia (benign). In these circumstances, the pathologist will usually seek the opinion of another (usually more experienced) pathologist. However, if he gets more than one opinion he may well receive more than one answer. If such a difficult case is circulated to ten or 20 experienced pathologists you can be almost guaranteed that a sizable proportion of them will disagree with the majority diagnosis. Pathologists frequently conduct such studies in all areas of pathology where diagnostic problems exist. These are interobserver studies and they serve to define and identify the extent and degree of diagnostic problems. The reason for such problems is that most biological processes form part of a continuum. In breast cancer, the continuum spreads from normal to hyperplasia, to atypical hyperplasia, to DCIS, to invasive cancer. Each of the five steps mentioned here is not a discrete step but consists of a dozen or more "substeps." In practice, most biopsies fall neatly into one of the categories above. The difficult diagnostic problems are difficult because they merge gently with one of the adjacent categories on the continuum. Think of it as being asked to distinguish between the various shades of gray. Everyone can distinguish between black and white. The average artist will readily distinguish between black and white and possibly three or five other shades of gray in between. As the number of shades increase, even an expert artist will begin to experience difficulty in distinguishing between them. The human eye, unlike a computer, cannot identify the 256 shades of gray present all around us. Nor can it identify the continuum of biological changes in a cell as it changes from benign to malignant.

At this stage, you may well be thinking—this is all very well as an intellectual game for pathologists, but what does it mean for the patient? It gets even more complicated. Consider, for example, a situation where a biopsy consists of four cores of breast tissue, each measuring 1 cm in length and 1 mm in diameter. More than 99 percent of the specimen show benign changes. However, at one edge of the specimen there is a single duct lined by atypical cells. Now, suppose that a highly experienced, highly expert pathologist decides, after much examination and deliberation, that the abnormality does not meet the required pathological criteria to make a diagnosis of malignancy and calls it atypical ductal hyperplasia. What should the surgeon do now? The significance of the change in the biopsy cannot be interpreted in isolation. What this means in practice is that these abnormalities must be interpreted in the light of other findings, in particular with those on the mammogram. Perhaps the biopsy hit an area just beside a more advanced abnormality, such as DCIS or invasive carcinoma. Such biopsy misses are sampling errors and depend on a combination of factors—the nature of the pathology, in particular the ratio of connective tissue stroma to epithelium, the number of samples taken, and the experience and expertise of the radiologist or surgeon taking the biopsy samples.

In difficult cases like this the pathologist, radiologist, and surgeon will, as a team, review the entire case. If they consider that there is a reasonable possibility of sampling error the surgeon will advise the patient to have another biopsy, possibly an excision biopsy, that is, excise the entire lump for pathological examination. As mentioned earlier we know from experience that such excisions after needle biopsy often reveal carcinoma. This type of team responsibility is now routine in most hospitals and is commonly called a "multidisciplinary approach" to patient care.

Unfortunately, most breast cancers present at a more advanced stage than DCIS; these are the invasive cancers. The usual breakdown on the ratio of DCIS to invasive carcinoma is 15 to 85 percent, and most of the DCIS are diagnosed in asymptomatic patients who chose to undergo routine screening mammography. Most patients with invasive breast cancer present with a painless lump.

The pathologic classification of invasive breast cancer is complicated (and frequently frustrates medical students the first time that they have to learn it). Invasive cancers are called invasive ductal or invasive lobular cancers, depending on their microscopic growth patterns. The distinction between them is not important. Far more important is the tumor grade, discussed below. Invasive carcinomas have subclassifications and some of these have an excellent prognosis. Most invasive ductal carcinomas are classified as "Invasive Breast Cancer, Not Otherwise Specified (NOS)." The others are grouped as cancers of a "specific type."

Invasive cancers have a basic structural similarity. Microscopically, they appear as sheets or groups of cells growing in an apparent random fashion in the breast stroma (the connective tissue framework in the breast). Although their overall appearance is broadly similar, they differ in subtle ways from each other. These subtle differences are sometimes important, as they often reveal biological secrets about their ability to metastasize and kill. It is these subtleties that pathologists use to grade cancer. Grade is a marker or indicator of a tumor's aggressiveness. Pathologists use three characteristics to grade invasive breast cancer: differentiation, pleomorphism, and mitoses.[2] It is important to note that this grading system is different from that used to grade DCIS.

Many cancers resemble normal ducts to varying degrees and this attempt to resemble normal tissue is called differentiation. In the breast, this means gland (duct) formation. The trained eye can easily identify differentiation. Pathologists also scrutinize the appearance of nuclei by comparing and contrasting them to normal nuclei and by comparing them to each other. Variation in nuclei from each other and their deviation from normal is called pleomorphism. The third important factor used to grade cancers is the number of mitoses present. Mitoses are dividing cells; when cells divide they multiply. So, the more mitoses present, the more rapidly the tumor is growing.

Each of these three parameters, differentiation, pleomorphism, and mitoses are scored from one to three and the final score gives the grade. Very well differentiated cancers get a score of one and undifferentiated cancers score three. Naturally, those in between score two. Likewise, there are scores of 1, 2, or 3 for pleomorphism and for mitoses. The final tally for any tumor can lie between 3 and 9. Tumors with scores of 3, 4, or 5 are low-grade tumors, those with a score of 6 or 7 are intermediate grade, and those scoring 8 or 9 are high grade. These are illustrated in Figure 4.5.

Tumor grade has proven itself as an important prognostic marker in numerous studies. Unfortunately, many doctors view grading with skepticism, as they regard it as too subjective and unreliable. The literature often seems to support these skeptics. Published studies indicate that in the past pathologists often showed considerable interobserver variability when asked to grade tumors precisely. A typical interobserver study includes a group of pathologists (often five or more). They study a set of slides prepared from, say, 50 tumors. Every pathologist places each tumor into a particular category, for example, benign, carcinoma in situ, and

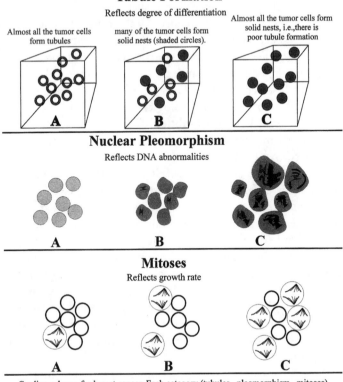

Tubule Formation

Reflects degree of differentiation

Almost all the tumor cells form tubules

many of the tumor cells form solid nests (shaded circles).

Almost all the tumor cells form solid nests, i.e.,there is poor tubule formation

A　　　**B**　　　**C**

Nuclear Pleomorphism

Reflects DNA abnormalities

A　　　**B**　　　**C**

Mitoses

Reflects growth rate

A　　　**B**　　　**C**

Grading scheme for breast cancer. Each category (tubules, pleomorphism, mitoses) gets 1 to 3 points (1 for A, 2 for B, 3 for C).

Scores for **low grade** tumors are 3, 4, and 5. Scores for **intermediate grade** tumors are 6, and 7. Scores for **high grade** tumors are 8 and 9.

Figure 4.5. Grading Scheme for Breast Cancer

invasive carcinoma, and grades the carcinomas as low, intermediate and high. Typically, such studies show the pathologists will almost always agree regarding the diagnosis (e.g., benign versus invasive carcinoma), but will disagree on the degree of abnormality (grade) within each category. There will be overlap between grade 1 and 2, and likewise between 2 and 3. Extreme disagreement (1 versus 3) is rare. The level of disagreement and overlap varies somewhat from study to study. The reliability of pathologic features other than diagnosis can be studied in a similar manner. For example, such studies show that blood vessel invasion cannot be identified accurately, consistently and reliably. In general, if a feature cannot be identified consistently, then it is unlikely to be a useful marker. Interobserver studies such as these are common in most branches of medicine and form part of the overall quality assurance imposed on medical doctors by their peers.

A careful, conscientious pathologist can easily grade breast cancer to a high standard. Advocates of grading have demonstrated that where pathologists are willing to learn the niceties of grading and take the time to apply them, they can do a good, reliable job. In recent years, the graders are winning. Newer studies confirm the value of grading and increasingly oncology protocols insist on grading. Despite the numerous new research techniques being applied to tumor tissue, grading is still a very valuable procedure and is one of the strongest prognostic predictors we have. Grading is important not just for breast cancers. It provides good prognostic information for many other cancers.

The "specific types" of invasive cancer appear to be less aggressive than the common cancers. It is important to recognize them, as they usually have an excellent prognosis. The more important ones are tubular carcinoma, mucinous (colloid) carcinoma, and papillary carcinoma. These are low-grade tumors with an excellent prognosis. More controversial is the medullary carcinoma. Paradoxically this is histologically a high-grade tumor but the medical literature claims that patients with these tumors have a better than average prognosis. These uncommon cancers show a florid infiltrate by lymphocytes (immune cells) and these may help destroy the tumor cells. Many experienced pathologists challenge this view and regard them as having the same prognosis as the "not otherwise specified" group of invasive ductal carcinomas.

Rarely, tumors other than these involve the breast either as primary tumors or as metastatic cancers to the breast. The primary tumors arise from the connective tissue surrounding the ducts and lobules. Liposarcomas arise from fat cells, fibrosarcomas arise from the fibroblasts (that produce collagen) and angiosarcomas arise from the cells that line the inner wall of blood vessels. Lymphomas can arise in the breast or spread from other organs.

The most common benign breast tumor is the fibroadenoma, mentioned above. This has a rare malignant counterpart—the phyllodes tumor (also called cystosarcoma phyllodes). This unusual tumor can behave as a low-grade or a high-grade tumor. Low-grade tumors do not metastasize and usually need only local removal and follow-up, whereas the high grade tumors often need a mastectomy.

The pathologist is almost always the final arbiter of whether a breast lump is benign or malignant. Accurate pathological assessment of every tumor is of critical importance. Not only does it give diagnostic information for the correct treatment, it also gives important prognostic information. The pathologist's report will state:

- the diagnosis
- the size of the tumor
- the grade of the tumor
- whether the surgical margins are free of tumor, and the distance between the nearest margin and the tumor
- whether there is any spread to lymph nodes, and if so how many nodes are involved
- whether the tumor cells are estrogen receptor positive or negative.

The oncologist will usually add Tamoxifen to the patient's treatment, if the tumor is estrogen receptor positive. Already some pathologists check to see if tumor cells are producing excessive amounts of the oncogene protein HER-2/neu. Some patients with this marker will benefit from treatment with Herceptin. As newer prognostic markers are identified, these will be added to the pathology report.

Mammography and Screening: The Key to Prevention?

What is a mammogram? It is an x-ray picture of the breast, taken with a specially designed machine. A trained radiographer takes two views of each breast, one from above and one from the side. She compresses each breast between two Plexiglas–like plates for a few seconds while the x-ray is being taken (Figure 5.1). Sometimes the compression is uncomfortable. However, compression is necessary as it flattens the breast tissue so that any tiny abnormalities will show up. A medically qualified radiologist interprets the findings.

Mammograms are used for two groups of women, those with breast symptoms and those without symptoms; thus the terminology, symptomatic mammography and screening mammography. The procedure takes about 20 minutes. In theory, mammography is simple; in practice, it is highly complicated, highly technical, and prone to numerous misunderstandings by the public, by administrators, and even by doctors.

A few fundamental facts about breast lumps and cancer will help us understand what we can expect of mammography.

- Some breast lumps are cancer; most are not.
- Most breast cancers produce lumps or some other symptoms; some do not.
- If a cancer contains denser tissue than surrounding normal breast, or if it contains calcium deposits, it will be visible on the mammogram.
- Not all abnormalities with calcium are cancer.
- All breast cancers are small before they are large, that is, large enough to be felt (or as doctors say, "palpable").
- Tumors may not be palpable if they are situated deep in a large breast.

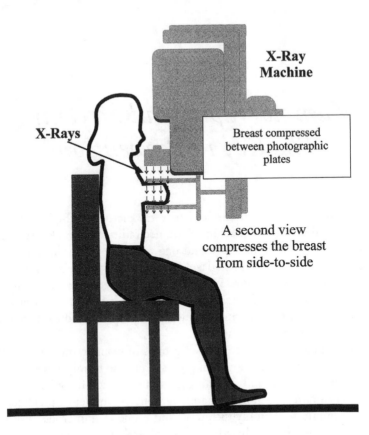

Figure 5.1. Mammogram

• Cancers about 0.5 cm are often visible on a mammogram. These cannot be palpated; they are too small.

• Mammograms can detect early cancer, either DCIS or small invasive tumors, before they are large enough to cause symptoms or become palpable.

• Mammograms can distinguish between cancerous lumps and non-cancerous lumps.

The main questions regarding this special technique are: (a) how reliably does mammography find cancer, and (b) how reliably does it distinguish cancer from benign abnormalities.

For any medical test to be useful, it has to have a high degree of "sensitivity" and a high degree of "specificity." The ideal test has 100 percent sensitivity and 100 percent specificity. This test would find every cancer and it would find only cancer; it would ignore every other abnormality. Such a test does not exist. In general, highly sensitive tests are usually not very specific, and highly specific tests are not very sensitive. So, doctors use a combination of tests to make a diagnosis; a highly sensitive test first, to find an abnormality, and then a highly specific test to diagnose the abnormality. The sensitive test picks up every abnormality. If it is negative, you can rest assured that it is normal. If it is positive, the abnormality may or may not be cancer. The obvious problem with a highly sensitive test is that it often produces "false positives." It detects too many abnormalities that are not cancer.

In contrast, a test with a high degree of specificity has few or no false positive results. Such tests are excellent diagnostic tests, but are often not very sensitive. They may ignore some abnormalities, and in so doing, miss some cancers.

Mammography falls short of the ideal test. It has numerous limitations, and some of these are discussed below. Although it is not perfect, it has a high level of sensitivity and specificity; while something better may come along in the future, it is the best screening test we have.

Although the value of a test is often measured in terms of sensitivity and specificity, other parameters, such as positive predictive and negative predictive values, give more useful information. These are derived from the sensitivity and specificity, and are discussed in an appendix at the end of this book. To find the value or usefulness of a screening test biostatisticians compare the results with a gold standard. For a positive test, they ask the question, "What are the chances that this abnormality is cancer?" In other words, what is the positive predictive value of a positive mammogram? Another way to ask this question is—if we have 100 women with a positive mammogram, what percentage of them has cancer? They need a gold standard to answer this question. The gold standard for a positive test is the biopsy.

For a negative test, the question is, "What are the chances that this woman does not have breast cancer if she has a negative mammogram?" Asked another way, it says, if we have 100 women with negative mammograms, how many of them have breast cancer? Obviously, if there is no abnormality on a mammogram, and there are no abnormal clinical findings, a biopsy is not indicated. Which part of the breast would you biopsy? Or, for that matter, which breast? So, the biopsy is not useful as a gold standard for a negative test. We need something else.

A true negative is indicated by the fact that no cancer appears after a period of follow-up. This period is usually two or three years, at which time a repeat mammogram is still negative. So, a negative mammogram followed two years later by another negative mammogram and no clinical signs of cancer is taken as a gold standard for "negative." Experts may disagree about the time scale one should wait but they agree in principle that some time scale should be used as a cut off line.

For individual patients, and for patients with any breast symptoms, doctors and cancer organizations recommend physical examination in addition to mammography. They recommend monthly self-examination and periodic examination by a health professional. However, in population screening programs physical examination does not provide any additional value to mammography (from a public health and statistical viewpoint). Most population screening programs do not include physical examination. Instead, they rely on the mammogram.

What Are the Limitations of a Mammogram?

In summary, the limitations of a mammogram are false positives, false negatives, and the consequences of these false results.

Because some cancers have a density similar to surrounding breast tissue, a mammogram can miss a tumor, even a large tumor that is clinically palpable. Some benign abnormalities are denser than surrounding normal breast and can mimic cancer. Calcium, one of the hallmarks of cancer in a mammogram, also finds its way into benign lesions. The ductal carcinoma in situ shown in figure 5.2 is easy to identify because of the extensive calcification; this would not present a challenge to any radiologist. However, often the changes are extremely subtle.

Let's look at the false negative rates first. A false negative means that the mammogram is reported as negative, when in fact the woman has cancer. We know she has cancer because sometime within the next one, two, or three years, she develops a cancerous lump, or a subsequent mammogram shows a cancer. Such cancers are called interval cancers. They arise during the interval between the initial and the subsequent examinations, or they were too small to be detected in the first mammogram, or the radiologist did not detect them. The definition of interval may vary from one screening program to another; most programs use two years as the cut off time. It is reasonable to expect more cancers to develop the longer you wait.

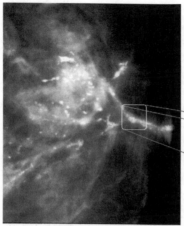

Mammogram showing extensive calcification within breast ducts.

The calcification occurs in the center of necrotic DCIS.

The white granular material is calcium.

DCIS showing such extensive involvement of many ducts (like here) will require mastectomy.

Breast-conserving surgery is usually not suitable when the disease is so widespread.

If pathology confirms that all the tumor cells are confined with the ducts (i.e., no invasive carcinoma) there is no risk of metastasis.

Figure 5.2. Ductal Carcinoma in Situ (DCIS)
(Mammogram courtesy Dr. Fidelma Flanagan)

What factors or variables contribute to a false negative mammogram? We can list the main factors as follows:

- the density of cancer and surrounding breast tissue
- a technically poor quality mammogram due to a poorly maintained x-ray machine
- a technically poor quality mammogram due to human error
- a poorly trained or inexperienced radiologist, or a highly trained radiologist who, for whatever reason, misses a subtle abnormality.

The nature of the cancer and the surrounding breast

Many cancers have an ill-defined outline and have a different x-ray density than the nearby breast tissue. Young breasts contain a lot of epithelium and fibrous stroma and relatively little fat (adipose tissue). In contrast, older breasts contain a lot of adipose tissue. The x-ray density of most cancers is very different from surrounding adipose tissue, so, in older breasts, dense cancers stand out from the surrounding breast tissue. However, in young breasts the density of the surrounding breast is very similar to that of cancer. This lack of contrast between the tumor and normal breast means that the tumor may not appear different from normal tissue, and produce a negative mammogram. This is one of the reasons why mammograms are less useful in young women. Some older women also have dense breast tissue, making cancer detection difficult. The other (more important) reason relates to the mathematics and statistics of prior probability, discussed in appendix A. Because of the rarity of cancer in young women, mammography is not so valuable as a screening tool in these women. I will discuss mammography for women in their 40s later in this chapter.

Equipment

The x-ray machine must be state-of-the-art mammographic equipment and maintained with the precision of a Formula-1 racing car. So too must the procedure for developing the radiographic films. Minor changes in such apparently trivial details as the temperature of the x-ray developing solutions will reduce radiographic sensitivity. Professional and hobbyist photographers who do their own darkroom work will appreciate this point. In comparison with modern mammographic units, earlier equipment was crude. It also delivered far more radiation to the breast. Modern equipment delivers tiny, safe doses of radiation.

The expertise of the personnel

Radiographers working in mammography units need special training. They need dedication and a commitment to meticulous detail. It helps also if they have warm, sympathetic personalities and good communication skills; these are the people who deal directly with the patients. ("Patients" is not a good term for women being screened, as these are perfectly normal women.)

Probably the most critical factor for quality screening is the skill and professional excellence of the people reading the mammograms, i.e., the radiologists. Radiologists are medically qualified doctors who subsequently specialize and become board certified in radiology. Not all board-certified radiologists are competent to interpret mammograms. The have additional specialist training devoted to mammography.

Radiology has become so diverse and sophisticated that it is impossible for any one person to become proficient in all areas of radiology, and to maintain proficiency. The interpretation of mammograms, especially those in asymptomatic women, is difficult. Mammograms in patients with palpable lumps are easier to interpret. Radiologists reading mammograms need special training, especially for screening mammography. This training allows them to become competent. However, the real problem is in maintaining competency. Unless a radiologist reports a large number (thousands) of mammograms each year the quality of reporting is likely to become substandard and the quality of the screening program will suffer. This means there will be too many false positive and false negative reports. This is most likely to happen in smaller hospitals or smaller screening units that do not have an adequate throughput of women to be screened, or in units that do not have radiologists and support staff dedicated to screening mammography.

What are the consequences of a false negative result? A false negative report will result in a delayed diagnosis—until a palpable lump appears, or a subsequent mammogram shows the abnormality—which may reduce the chance of cure. Furthermore, the option for breast-conserving surgery may be lost. Ductal carcinoma in situ (DCIS) and small invasive cancers usually need less surgery, i.e., they often do not need a mastectomy. DCIS patients do not need chemotherapy, whereas patients with more advanced cancers often do. The rationale for screening is to identify in situ and small cancers. These cancers are curable and have no risk, or a low-risk, of metastasizing. They also allow the woman to have breast-conserving surgery, rather than mastectomy. An exception to this is the unusual situation where in situ carcinoma involves many different parts of the breast.

The usual cause of a false negative report is that, for whatever reason, the radiologist misses an abnormality in the mammogram. The radiologist depends on the person making the mammogram, i.e., the radiographer, to produce an excellent quality x-ray. In turn, the radiographer relies on well-maintained high-quality x-ray equipment. Poor quality mammograms lead the radiologist to the wrong conclusion, resulting in a wrong report. A weak link anywhere will break the chain of excellence needed for a high-quality screening program. Even if a mammogram is technically excellent, an interruption or a momentary lapse of concentration can cause a radiologist to miss a minor (but significant) abnormality.

As in all occupations, even the best, most dedicated and conscientious radiologists will make occasional mistakes. These are rarely mistakes of negligence. Reading dozens of normal mammograms at a single reporting session can become tiring. Radiologists often devise strategies to minimize distractions. In order to maintain a high level of concentration, they randomly add mammograms with known subtle abnormalities to their routine workload. By doing this they heighten their anticipation of an impending abnormality. This keeps them focused on the task at hand. Some radiologists devise strategies and techniques that force them to examine each segment or each breast in a piecemeal, methodological fashion. The knowledge that their reports are possibly going to be scrutinized by inspectors (not to mention hungry attorneys) also helps to keep them concentrating. It is a tough job. New computer programs help radiologists focus on the correct areas of a mammogram by detecting and highlighting areas of potential abnormalities. The idea is to draw the radiologist's attention to subtle abnormalities that could be overlooked.

To further reduce the false negatives, many programs use double reading. Two radiologists read each set of mammograms independently. This reduces the chance of overlooking minor abnormalities missed by one human expert, who for whatever reason might be distracted during the examination. Most programs now also add additional mammographic views of each breast. This is called double view mammography, and it too helps to reduce the false negatives.

For more than a decade, high-technology companies have struggled with the idea of teaching computers to read mammograms, and they have made tremendous progress. The idea is to scan the mammogram into a computer where special digital imaging software recognizes and classifies abnormalities.[1-3] The computer is trained to mimic how the human reads and interprets a mammogram. The human eye-brain combination is still far better than a scanner and computer. Nevertheless, experts in the fields of mammography and computer technology are confident that in the near future computers will replace some of the radiologist's work. In November 2000 the U.S. Food and Drug Administration approved the first complete digital mammogram system, and so far 75 digital machines have been installed in the U.S.

Computers have made analogous conquests in other areas of high cerebral activity. For example, the modern computer program "Deep Blue" is more than a worthy match for most chess grand masters, as it demonstrated by beating world champion Garry Kasparov in 1997. Also, computers now detect cervical cancer. Computers can screen cervical cytology slides with a high degree of accuracy. The FDA has approved automated (computerized) cytology systems to improve cervical cytology screening in certain circumstances. A computer at the end of a microscope decides whether cervical cells are abnormal or not. That is its sole function, and it does it well. Once it detects an abnormality the pathologist takes over and makes the definitive diagnosis.

Likewise, the hope for radiologists is that their system will be good enough to separate normal from abnormal. Already, some university centers are testing these systems and expect to have them in clinical use before the year 2005.

Even if the radiologist spots a suspicious abnormality, the final conclusion may be a false negative report. Consider the situation where a radiologist sees an abnormality and thinks it is an area suspicious for malignancy, but has some doubts about the diagnosis. Under such circumstances, after reviewing the mammograms with colleagues and possibly taking new mammograms, he or she places a fine needle into the abnormality and aspirates cells for the pathologist to examine. The radiologist guides the needle into the abnormal area using computerized guiding equipment (stereotactic biopsy) or sophisticated ultrasound equipment. Even if the abnormality on the x-ray is malignant, the aspirated specimen may contain too few cells to make a diagnosis, or it may consist of benign cells, which lie beside tumor cells. This situation also gives a false negative diagnosis. There are even more pitfalls; these lie at the microscope. Like the radiologist, the pathologist needs special training and competence in interpreting breast cytology. Even a well-trained, competent pathologist may fail to diagnose subtle cellular changes indicative of malignancy.

How often do false negatives like this occur? Not very often in a good screening unit. It is difficult to give precise figures. However, because cytology has too many false negative results in some screening units, there is a worldwide trend towards abandoning fine needle breast cytology in favor of needle core biopsies. These obtain small fragments of tissue rather than just cells, and, in general, are easier to interpret than cytology specimens. Furthermore, the new biopsy guns cause no more patient discomfort than fine needle aspiration. Despite the trend towards biopsy, many units claim they get results just as good with needle aspiration.

What are consequences of a false positive mammogram? First, we need to define what exactly is a false positive. Different studies use different definitions. The most radical definition would be mastectomy for a radiographic abnormality in the mistaken belief that it was cancer.

Thirty years ago, some surgeons performed mastectomies for lumps that appeared clinically malignant. In most cases, the clinical diagnosis was correct. However, sometimes they got it wrong and the unfortunate woman lost a breast unnecessarily. To the best of my knowledge mastectomy without a prior biopsy diagnosis no longer happens. In Western countries, such a practice is unthinkable.

When the era of mammography first arrived, unnecessary mastectomies resulted from incorrectly interpreted mammograms. More commonly, surgeons removed just the abnormal area for pathologic diagnosis. This is an excision biopsy. Sometimes the abnormality was benign and the mammogram was classified as a false positive. Although this procedure seems relatively minor in comparison to mastectomy, the biopsy sometimes removes a large part of the breast. Clearly, in most circumstances, it is unacceptable to remove a large portion of breast for benign disease.

As radiologists became more expert, and their equipment became more sophisticated, they began to make preoperative diagnoses using fine needle aspiration of mammographic abnormalities. Despite the painful image you might have of a long needle penetrating deep into a woman's breast, for most patients this is a trivial medical procedure and is not as uncomfortable as the breast compression required to take the mammogram. As explained above, there is a trend towards using needle core biopsies rather than needle aspiration to make the final diagnosis. If any procedure removes tissue or cells and these do not show cancer, the mammogram that led to the procedure is classified as false positive.

Recent studies broaden the definition of "positive." They include any abnormal mammogram where the woman does not have cancer, even if she does not have an invasive procedure. For example, some women require a second-look mammogram to better define an area of minor or borderline abnormality. This procedure might be a repeat mammogram for a technically poor original mammogram, or a magnified view of a specific area, or an ultrasound examination to distinguish a cyst from a fibroadenoma. Using broad criteria like these, Dr. Elmore, from the University of Washington School of Medicine, found over a period of ten years that one third of women screened had an abnormal test that needed additional evaluation.[4,5] Most radiologists would argue that these are not false positive mammograms as no invasive procedure was performed. These additional tests are performed to clarify equivocal changes in the first mammogram. To classify such as a "false positive" seems pedantic. However, some experts classify any abnormality that leads to another procedure as a false positive. Their argument is that every procedure, no matter how minor, leads to anxiety; sometimes the anxiety and fear is overwhelming.[6]

Quality Assurance (QA)

Program directors, organizers, surgeons, and radiologists, conscious of the physical and psychological insults of false positives and false negatives, try to keep these to a minimum. However, in doing so, screening inevitably misses some cancers, and overcalls others. As mentioned above mammography is not perfect. Nevertheless, screeners now have the benefit of 30 years worldwide experience and they know the pitfalls and they know how to minimize false results. Centers of excellence use the information gathered over the years to help them give a quality service. If you decide to have a mammogram, have it done at a center of excellence.[7]

How can you recognize a center of excellence? A center of excellence will have a quality assurance (QA) program that monitors every minute detail of the program, from the quality of the x-ray development through to the final pathology report (if there is pathology). It monitors the ratio of benign to malignant biopsies. Too high a ratio (i.e., too many false positives) indicates that the radiologists are overcalling too many subtle changes. It monitors how quickly the reports get back to family doctors and patients, and it monitors how the information is conveyed in the report.

An excellent program with rigorous quality assurance checks the sensitivity of all its equipment on a daily or weekly basis. You might wonder how it can do this. Radiologists use a phantom test.

This test uses a plastic block, representing an average-sized compressed breast. It contains wax inserts that hold 16 test objects: six fibrous structures (fibers), five embedded microcalcifications (speck groups), and five different sized tumor-like masses that simulate tumors. The numbers that show up on the test mammogram determine the quality of the mammographic image.

QA programs ensure that all its professionals participate in regular continuous medical education and regular self-assessment exercises. It insists that surgeons, radiologists, and pathologists meet regularly to discuss and make decisions about difficult and problem cases. These are called triple assessment conferences. In addition, it records all its activities and results and makes this information available for scrutiny by outside inspection teams. Such rigorous quality assurance allows the organizers to compare their results with those from other national and international programs. An excellent program will be proud of its work and will probably publish these figures in an annual report.

If problems arise with any aspect of quality assurance, the program directors and managers must take remedial action. If performance falls below accepted standards, they, or outside regulating bodies, have the power to stop screening and close down the program. Poor breast screening is worse than no screening.

How will you know if the center is keeping up to speed with all these parameters? You will not know the details, but in the United States the center will have an FDA–approved certificate displayed in a prominent position. The precise details of quality assurance may vary slightly in other countries. However, wherever there are government-sponsored screening programs there will be rigorous quality assurance.

The Mammography Quality Standards Act of 1992 (MQSA) in the U.S. ensures high quality mammography in certified mammography centers. This act requires all mammography centers (10,000 in the U.S.) to meet quality assurance criteria for equipment, safety, personnel qualifications, image quality, and practices. Before this act took effect, 11 percent of facilities tested failed image quality tests; recent figures were less than two percent and improving. The standards are based primarily on those recommended by the American College of Radiology (ACR). Centers not complying with regulations are fined or shut down. In November 1997, organizers, and ultimately legislators, recognized that a particular unit in the U.K. was performing poorly. The government closed the unit. Likewise, U.S. officials have closed or fined units not complying with MQSA regulations.

The act also requires accreditation and each facility must have an annual inspection by FDA–approved inspectors. New legislation controlling quality assurance in mammography has ensured proficiency in almost all hospitals and clinics with mammography services.[7]

The National Cancer Institute has a Mammography Information Service line at 1-800-422-6237 (TTY: 1-800-332-8615) that will provide a list of certified mammography facilities in your geographic area. NCI also provides excellent information at its main web site at www.nci.nih.gov. You can obtain information from your local American Cancer Society chapters by calling 1-800-227-2345.

While not certified under MQSA, Veterans Administration (VA) facilities operate under a similar program. For information about VA facilities, call their Mammography Help Line at 1-888-492-7844. Information on Food and Drug Administration (FDA) mammography sites are here: http://www.ntis.gov/fcpc/cpn7336.htm.

Some European countries, notably Sweden, the Netherlands, and United Kingdom, have national breast screening programs, and their quality assurance criteria are just as rigorous (and possibly even more strict) than U.S. criteria. They invite their entire population of women between the ages of 50 and 65 (and sometimes older) for screening. Such programs have enormous, and at times overwhelming, managerial problems. Other European countries, Canada, and Australia are either in the process of setting up, or have recently set up, national and regional programs.

Pathologists use similar safeguards to ensure that their diagnoses are accurate. In the U.K., almost 600 pathologists subject their work to scrutiny by their peers twice every year. Their level of accuracy is compared to that of an expert group of 20 pathologists. An expert group from European countries subject themselves to similar quality assurance exercises.

Surgeons have quality assurance programs to ensure that they carry out the most appropriate surgery. They ask questions such as, are the biopsy margins around a cancer clear and by how much (confirmed by pathology)? Is the amount of breast tissue removed for a 1 cm cancer appropriate, too much, or too little (they quantify the amount of tissue by weighing and measuring it)? Is the mastectomy rate in this program too high, too low, or just right? Is the recurrence rate after surgery acceptable (in comparison with other centers that are doing a good job)? Is the amount of tissue removed for the diagnosis of a benign lesion appropriate? Are the post-operative recovery rates and the complication rates acceptable by international standards?

Quality assurance does not stop with radiologists, surgeons, and pathologists. It encompasses the work of physicists calibrating equipment, radiographers performing the mammograms, epidemiologists and biostatisticians monitoring results, and other support staff logging thousands of data items. It concerns the laboratory technicians striving to make excellent quality cytology and tissue preparations. All these strategies and procedures help maintain the overall quality assurance of the program, and quality assurance procedure manuals record these procedures.

Does Screening Work?

Critics will say "screening doesn't work," or at least the case is unproven. There is often confusion about what is meant by "screening." When they say it doesn't work, what they mean is that the program does not reduce the overall mortality in the population (region, country or whatever). They quote old or poorly implemented studies. One of the reasons some programs do not work is that many women do not use the facility. Unless approximately 70 percent of the women invited take up the offer, the "program" will fail to show an overall reduction in mortality. This then is interpreted as proving that "screening doesn't work." With a small number of exceptions, it works for the women who are screened.

It also works for the population, provided the program enforces strict quality assurance on all parts of the program, and approximately 70 percent of the population participates. Where screening is carried out systematically and carefully, experts say we can achieve a 20 to 25 percent reduction in mortality from breast cancer.[8] Additional bonuses for detecting early breast cancer are less surgery, better morale, and lower treatment costs.

Is regular screening necessary for all women? Scientists, politicians, and women's advocacy groups differ radically on the value of mammography screening for women in their 40s.[9] There is no argument about women in high-risk groups, especially those with strong family histories. All agree that screening benefits high-risk groups. The debate focuses on women with normal risks in their 40s. Proponents argue that screening saves lives, and that it is wrong to withhold screening in this age group. Opponents argue that cancers are uncommon in this age group, they are more difficult to find, there are too many false positives, and that screening does more harm than good. They say that large numbers of women without cancer but with minor mammographic abnormalities undergo unnecessary biopsies. Experts estimate that one million U.S. women in their 40s have false positive mammograms every year. One study found false-positive results produced short-term psychological troubles, such as anxiety, distress, and intrusive thoughts. Sometimes the distress lasted up to 18 months.[6]

On January 23, 1997, an advisory panel of the National Cancer Institute, after a detailed examination, decided that there was not sufficient proof to recommend screening for women in their 40s. They suggested that screening in this age group should be left to the discretion of doctors and the wishes of individual women. During the following weeks, outraged politicians, doctors, and patients voiced their disagreement. On March 27, the NCI reversed its decision and recommended screening for these women. Many observers felt they had given in to the politicians and ignored scientific facts. Dr. Jane Wells of the Institute of Health Sciences at the University of Oxford, U.K., writing in the British Medical Journal critically of the NCI reversed decision, concludes, "When trials do not give an unequivocal answer, when politicians and interest groups become involved, and when the professionals responsible for promoting the public's best interest fail to do so, objectivity is likely to suffer."[10] This, it seems, is what happened with the decision to screen women in their 40s.

The facts suggest that the case for screening young women is unproven. However, there is deep disagreement among cancer specialists. The American Cancer Society and the American College of Radiology believe that screening for younger women is beneficial. The crux of the matter is that neither scientists nor doctors know for sure. Statisticians calculate that in order to answer the question, approximately 450,000 women would have to be enrolled in a mammography study. This is not practical, and many would argue that it is not ethical. One statistical model estimated that if 10,000 women in their 40s underwent mammography, four would live longer. Against this, 3,000 women without cancer would have had a mammogram interpreted as abnormal (false positives), and many of these would have needed a biopsy.

Using cost analysis figures, advocates argue that screening for women in their 40s is extremely cost-effective. They argue that it is more cost-effective than annual Pap screening for cervical cancer or seat belts and air bags in cars. Dr. Stephen A. Feig, director of the Breast Imaging Center at Thomas Jefferson University in Philadelphia, Pennsylvania, told delegates at a meeting in Boston that annual screening for women in their 40s cost $9,000 per year of life saved (in 1999) (Source: ReutersHealth). In contrast, the annual cost of cervical cancer screening is $12,000 per year of life saved and seat belts and air bags cost $32,000 per year of life saved. I must confess that I have no idea how these figures were arrived at.

Despite the conflicts and arguments, there is overwhelming agreement that screening, if done properly, is beneficial to women after the age of 50 and is beneficial to some women before the age of 50. U.S. agencies advise mammography every one or two years, beginning at the age of 40, and annually after age 50. European agencies advise women after the age of 50 to have a mammogram every two years. The American Cancer Society also advises women to begin monthly self-examination in their 20s. They also advise them to have a clinical examination by a healthcare professional every three years. After the age of 40, the clinical examination should be every two years, and after the age of 50, every year.

Is mammography the key to prevention? Unfortunately, no. The Pap smear detects cellular abnormalities in the cervix before they become cancerous; regular Pap smears can prevent cancer. Mammography cannot make similar claims. It cannot detect changes before they become malignant. However, because it detects early and small cancers, it can prevent premature death from breast cancer, if used appropriately.

Hereditary Breast Cancer: Looking for Clues in DNA

Cancer often appears to run in families. Some malignancies are inherited through faulty genes. However, because cancer is so common, it is not unusual for a number of family members to get cancer purely by statistical coincidence. This is called chance aggregation.

Shared exposure to an environmental carcinogen is another possible explanation for multiple cancer victims in a family. For example, multiple members of the same family might get cancer because they work in the shipbuilding industry and are exposed to asbestos. Workers exposed to asbestos, dioxin, polyvinyl chloride, and many other chemicals in their environment are at risk for various cancers. These chemicals enter the cell and mutate the genes responsible for cell growth. Sometimes the damage comes from what we eat, drink, or inhale. For breast cancer there is no known environmental carcinogen, although many experts believe dietary factors are at least partly responsible.

Genetic mutations, inherited from one or both of our parents, also cause cancer. This is hereditary or familial cancer.

So, we can think of cancer as having two major causes: a hereditary tendency and the environment. For some cancers the hereditary component is overwhelming and far more important than any environmental toxins. Familial Adenomatosis Polyposis (FAP) is one well-known example. In this disease, thousands of neoplastic polyps sit in the large intestine, like tiny time bombs. If they are not removed, they turn into lethal malignant tumors. Children inherit this disease from one of the parents through a genetic mutation on the long arm of chromosome 5. Unless they have major surgery they will have colon cancer in their 20s or 30s. Other examples of hereditary cancers include some forms of Wilms' tumor in children (kidney), familial renal cancer (kidney), and retinoblastoma (eye).

Some breast cancers are hereditary. Typically, familial breast cancer affects a woman in her 30s or 40s, whose mother also had breast cancer at a young age. Her sisters are also at risk. Many of these women, and their sisters and daughters, are also at risk for ovarian cancer. Approximately ten percent of breast cancers are familial. A tiny number strike patients with known hereditary syndromes such as the Li-Fraumeni syndrome, Ataxia Telangiectasia, and Cowden's syndrome.[1,2] In the Li-Fraumeni syndrome, inherited mutations of the p53 gene cause cancer in many different organs. These include soft tissue sarcomas, brain tumors, leukemia, and breast cancer.[3-6] Patients with Ataxia-telangiectasia are also at risk for leukemia. Cowden's syndrome is a combination of intestinal polyps and benign tumors of the skin and uterus.[7] The mutated genes for these rare diseases have been discovered recently.[8] Some studies question whether the inherited genetic damage is the main cause of breast cancer in Cowden's syndrome. Other genes may also play a role.[9]

Although the above genetic disorders are recent entries in the medical literature, for almost 100 years experienced clinicians knew that some breast cancers were hereditary. During the past 20 years, scientists armed with new molecular techniques have hunted for breast cancer genes. In 1994, researchers found the BRCA1 gene.[10,11] It is a tumor suppresser gene whose exact function is unknown. BRCA1 sits on the long arm of chromosome 17 (17q21), close to a number of other genes implicated in cancer progression and aggressiveness. These include HER-2/neu and p53. BRCA1, like other suppresser genes, helps control orderly cell growth. Mutations in this gene are common in hereditary breast cancer but are rare in sporadic breast cancer.

Shortly after the discovery of BRCA1, scientists found the BRCA 2 gene.[12] BRCA2 is located on the long arm of chromosome 13[13] and its function is to fix broken DNA. Scientists call it a "caretaker" gene. Caretaker genes monitor the cell cycle and repair errors as they occur. Together, BRCA1 and BRCA2 mutations account for approximately 50 percent of familial breast cancers. This means that they account for approximately five percent of all breast cancers. The genes responsible for the other hereditary cancers remain unknown.

The influence of a mutated BRCA1 or BRCA2 is powerful. Early reports indicated that women with a family history of breast cancer and mutated BRCA1 had an 80 to 90 percent chance of developing breast cancer. More recent studies suggest that in the absence of a clear-cut family history BRCA1 mutations confer a much lower risk—in the region of 57 percent. Furthermore, these women have a 16 percent risk for ovarian cancer. It appears that certain genetically related racial groups, such as

Ashkenazi Jews, have a high incidence of BRCA1 and BRCA2 mutations. The Ashkenazis originate from central Europe and they make up over 90 percent of the Jewish population living in the United States. One in every 100 Ashkenazi women has a mutated BRCA2. Some authorities estimate that up to 1 in 50 (two percent) have a mutation in either BRCA1 or BRCA2. Clearly, factors other than a mutated BRCA contribute to familial breast cancer, but how these additional variables influence the affect of the mutations is unknown.

New molecular biology techniques make testing for BRCA1 and BRCA2 mutations possible. At present, experts suggest that the following women should be screened for BRCA1 and BRCA2 mutations:

1. Closely related women with breast or ovarian cancer—mother, daughter, sister.
2. Patients with premenopausal breast cancer.
3. Patients with breast cancer under the age of 40 (or possibly even under 50).
4. Patients with breast and ovarian cancer.
5. Patients with bilateral breast cancer.
6. Ashkenazi Jewish women.

However, whether these tests should be offered to women without a family history is a hotly debated issue. The significance of a positive test in the absence of family history is unknown. One eminent scientist described our current attempts at predicting the future for women having these tests as like "fortune-telling with a cloudy crystal ball."

Those who recommend more liberal use of genetic screening tests argue that positive results allow more aggressive surveillance and early treatment. Better surveillance, with more frequent physical examinations and mammography at a younger age, should identify the first signs of cancer. They argue that genetic testing ought to be part of a continuum of cancer management, and that it would allow women with a positive test to make more informed choices.

Recent research provides conflicting information for patients with familial breast cancer, regarding prognosis. Some studies claim they have a better long-term prognosis than patients with nonfamilial cancers.[14,15] The reason for this is unclear. One possible explanation is that these tumors are less aggressive. Another possible reason is that patients with familial cancer are screened and diagnosed at an earlier stage, and treated more aggressively. Conflicting results come from other studies that show that the prognosis is worse,[16] or not different from patients with nonfamilial cancers.[17]

Many authorities feel that widespread testing is premature. The main problem with a positive test is that, at present, it is unclear what is the best way to act on such a result. What to do if the test is positive for mutations is unclear. Similarly, a negative test does not guarantee that the woman will not get cancer.

Theoretical statistical models try to predict survival after prophylactic surgery. One study hypothesizes that if a 30-year-old woman with a BRCA1 or BRCA2 mutation has both breasts removed prophylactically, she can expect a gain in her life span of three to five years. Removal of her ovaries would result in a gain of four to 20 months.[18] The poor gain for oophorectomy is partly due to an increased risk for coronary artery disease and heart failure. In contrast to this model, a similar calculation for a woman over the age 60 shows that prophylactic breast surgery adds less than one year to her life span. Despite these gloomy predictions, some women seek prophylactic bilateral mastectomies. The usual operation is subcutaneous mastectomy. This operation does not guarantee a woman freedom from breast cancer. Tiny groups of breast glands may remain embedded in the tissue beneath the preserved nipple[19] and these can become malignant.

Luckily, facts do not always support theories. New encouraging studies from Columbia University in New York and from the Mayo Clinic indicate that bilateral prophylactic mastectomy is protective. These studies show that the risk for women with a family history is reduced by 90 percent.[20-22] Another possible piece of good news is the evidence that the birth control pill can reduce the risk of ovarian cancer in patients with BRCA1 and BRCA2 mutations. One study shows a 60 percent risk reduction in women using oral contraceptives for six or more years.[23] Before we get enthusiastic about information such as this, we need confirmation from more studies.

Many questions remain unanswered regarding BRCA1 and BRCA2 mutations. These large genes have complex structures, and mutations hit different parts of the gene. To date, over 200 mutations have been identified in BRCA1.[24] It is too early to state whether all these mutations carry the same clinical significance or the same risk for cancer. Emerging data suggest that some mutations are more important than others.[25-29]

How well the nation's laboratories can accurately identify precise mutations is unknown. Only a small number of laboratories provide the service. The National Cancer Institute has set up a national genetics network to address unresolved questions regarding accuracy of testing, implications of different mutations, and their significance in the absence of a strong family history. They also provide education for health care professionals and advise them about best counseling procedures.[30]

Together, computer and biology scientists have created the "gene chip." This may overcome many of the shortcomings in testing for mutations. At present, conventional tests must target specific mutations. These tests look at either the few most common mutation areas on the gene, or in the case of families with known mutations, at a previously identified mutation. Current tests use gel technology and automated gene sequencing and take days of laboratory time to perform. The newer gene chips will identify all the mutations, located anywhere on a gene. They will analyze the entire range of genetic mutations, in hours, rather than days. Already, preliminary trials for BRCA1 mutations have shown great promise. The gene chip acts like a word processing spell-check. It identifies mismatched letters of the genetic alphabet, and flags them for the geneticist to verify the result.

Who can have their BRCA genes examined? In the U.S., anyone willing to pay the commercial price of about $2,000 (in 1999). This price will undoubtedly drop in a few years. In the U.K., anyone who falls into an accepted risk category can have it for free. Their doctors will insist that they have appropriate counseling before they are tested. The rules and opportunities vary from country to country. Cancer specialists and geneticists and their representative professional bodies are adamant that this test should not be made available to the general public. There are too many unanswered questions. It is just not possible yet to advise the public how best they should respond to a positive or negative test. Often, testing is carried out as part of a clinical trial. These patients are guaranteed confidentiality and expert medical, genetic, and psychological counseling.

Many groups in society have serious concerns about genetic screening. Geneticists, ethicists, and sociologists argue that widespread genetic screening would provide inappropriate information for insurance companies. With bad-risk information they could load premiums or deny insurance coverage.[31,32] Genetic information on an individual may come from new genetic tests or from the results of genetic tests already in a patient's medical record. These may have been performed sometime in the past. Even if a patient never had genetic tests, her medical record may contain important genetic information derived from a family history.

Insurance companies are interested in two major areas relating to genetics. These are healthcare and life insurance. The relative problems in these areas vary in different countries. For example, in the U.K., the government's National Health Service covers most of the population for all healthcare, and an appropriate budget covers medical care due to genetic diseases. However, in the U.S., a large proportion of the population is covered by private insurance. Private insurance companies in every country are deeply concerned about the impact genetic information may have on their earnings. Knowledge about high-risk groups would help them reduce their payouts. They are also concerned about their relationships with governments, national and international genetic organizations, and the public, and are ready to do battle.

In the U.K., the Association of British Insurers (ABI) believes there are eight genetic disorders which insurers would like to know about; three of them are cancers. These are Familial Adenomatous Polyposis (which leads to colon cancer), multiple endocrine neoplasia (thyroid, parathyroid, adrenal and other cancers), and hereditary breast cancer. The others are Huntington's disease, myotonic dystrophy, hereditary motor and sensory neuropathy, some forms of Alzheimer's disease, and polycystic kidney disease. According to a British advisory group, the Human Genetics Advisory Commission (HGAC), insurers should have no access to genetic information. On the other side of the argument, insurers worry that individuals who have private genetic information might be tempted to stock up on their life insurance.

In the U.S., the National Institutes of Health (NIH) in conjunction with other respected and influential bodies recommends that insurance companies should not use genetic information to deny insurance coverage, to reduce coverage, or to increase premiums. The American Medical Association (AMA) and its 300,000 members endorse these views. Employing agencies could also discriminate on the basis of a genetic test that indicated you were at risk for developing breast cancer, or some other cancer, or for that matter, any other disease. Many individuals feel they are denied jobs or discriminated against because they have a genetic disorder. In one U.S. study in 1996, 22 percent of those surveyed believed they were denied healthcare insurance because they had a genetic disorder.

More than 30 U.S. states have already passed laws prohibiting genetic tests on job applicants. The Equal Opportunity Commission believes that discrimination based on genetic information contravenes the Americans with Disabilities Act. New legislation such as the Health Insurance Portability and Accountability Act (U.S. 1996) may provide adequate protection against abusive genetic information.

Until recently, many commentators felt that genetic testing was premature,[33] because patients, doctors and counselors did not know how to act on the results of genetic tests. Information on breast cancer is accruing quicker than for most other cancers. In the year 2001, muddy waters are beginning to clear. It is likely to take another decade before we have widely accepted guidelines for genetic screening for many types of cancer.[34-36]

Diagnosis: How Doctors Decide What a Breast Lump Is

When a woman discovers a breast lump, panic strikes. She immediately thinks the worst. She remembers stories she has read or seen in TV documentaries about the horrors of cancer and chemotherapy. She may recall relatives, friends, or neighbors who have died of breast or other cancers. Some women will not have this reaction and will ignore it and do nothing about it. Most will end up trembling in their doctor's office demanding to know just one thing: Is it cancer?

A brief interview will probe relevant questions. How long has it been there? Has it grown during this time? If so, by how much? Is it painful or sore? Have you found any other lumps in the breast, the other breast, under the arm or elsewhere? Are there any other breast symptoms? The doctor will also probe the family history to see if any close relatives had breast cancer, and if so at what age.

The Examination

Unlike the many and varied symptoms that come with disorders of other organs, symptoms of breast disease are few. A woman may visit her doctor for such reasons as:

• No symptoms—routine check-up or mammogram
• Lump
• Pain
• Nipple discharge

- Nipple soreness, or soreness of surrounding skin
- Skin changes away from the nipple
- Symptoms or signs due to metastases (back pain, epilepsy, general fatigue).

Breast cancer may produce no symptoms, or any one, or any combination of the above symptoms. Each symptom is non-specific. Put another way, no symptom is diagnostic of cancer and benign conditions can produce any of these symptoms.

No symptoms

Early breast cancer produces no symptoms, and radiologists, using mammography, can detect abnormalities long before there are any symptoms. Increasingly, breast cancers are being detected in asymptomatic women. This is encouraging, as most of these women are curable.

Lump

A lump is by far the most common symptom (Figure 7.1). Most lumps are caused by one of the following: fibroadenoma, a simple cyst, fibrocystic disease, or carcinoma. Normal breasts often have a generalized lumpi-

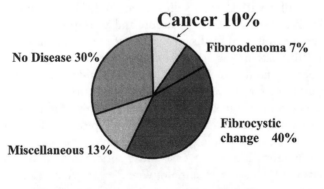

Cancer 10%

No Disease 30%

Fibroadenoma 7%

Fibrocystic change   40%

Miscellaneous 13%

Final results in women attending clinic for apparent lumps (1,000 women of all ages).

(Adapted from Ellis H, Cox PJ. Postgraduate Medical Journal, 1984)

Figure 7.1. Breast Lumps

ness. Patients with diffusely lumpy, bumpy breasts need only reassurance (possibly after a mammogram). A real lump may be obvious or so subtle that the woman is not sure she has a lump at all. Sometimes, a family doctor may be equally unsure. If the family doctor confirms that a lump is present, or is suspicious that one might be present, he or she will often refer the patient to a surgeon for more definitive diagnosis. With some benign lumps, the diagnosis is immediately obvious and a biopsy may not be necessary.

Fibroadenomas often have characteristic findings. They are usually pea-sized, but size is variable and they can be smaller or larger. What distinguishes them from other breast abnormalities is the way they move freely within the breast tissue. When an examining finger is placed on top of the lump, the fibroadenoma slips away. In medical jargon, it is freely mobile. When a woman in her 20s finds a breast lump, it is usually a fibroadenoma. Cancer in this age group is remarkably rare. These typical findings in fibroadenoma are not always present. Sometimes, it is embedded tightly in dense breast tissue and is unable to move about. If it calcifies it may feel harder than usual. Because fibroadenomas are not malignant or premalignant, there is no need to remove them. Nevertheless, surgeons often remove a fibroadenoma because the woman feels it is safer to have it out. If there is any doubt or query about the diagnosis the surgeon will recommend removal. If found incidentally in a mammogram they are often left undisturbed.

Like a fibroadenoma, a cyst is round and distinct from surrounding tissue. It is filled with slightly yellow clear fluid. The doctor can confirm the lesion is a cyst by inserting a needle and aspirating fluid.[1] Clear fluid in the syringe, followed by disappearance of the lump, reassures the surgeon and the patient that the lesion is a cyst. Bloodstained or cloudy, dirty appearing fluid is an indication that it should be sent to the pathology department for cytological examination. If the lump remains, or if it is not a cyst, the surgeon is likely to insert a fine needle into the lump to aspirate cells. This is termed fine needle aspiration (FNA) cytology. Alternatively he may decide to biopsy the abnormality. Another way to tell the difference between a cyst and a solid tumor is by ultrasound examination.[2,3] This uses technology similar to what is used in sonar equipment in submarines and can readily distinguish between solid tissue and a cyst.

Fibrocystic disease (FCD) is one of the most common conditions to cause a lump. The lump may be subtle or obvious, and it may occupy one part of the breast or multiple areas—in one or both breasts. An experienced surgeon can usually tell the difference between fibrocystic disease and cancer. However, in a middle-aged woman, the surgeon will often, justifiably, order a mammogram to add confidence to the benign diagnosis.

A small breast cancer produces no symptoms. It grows silently usually for many years before drawing attention to itself. When it does so, its symptoms depend on a number of factors—its location, its size, the size of the breast, and whether or not it involves the overlying skin or nipple.

Cancerous lumps can be small or large, soft or hard, painful or nonpainful. Mostly they are not painful. Whether they are small or large depends on their stage at the time of discovery. Occasionally, a woman will find a lump in the armpit as the first indicator of breast cancer. Rarely, a patient may present with symptoms that initially appear totally unrelated to the breast. For example, a fractured hip or back pain due to metastases may be the presenting complaint.

Pain

Breast pain can vary from ill-defined discomfort to searing pangs. The most common breast pains are due to hormones. These cause cyclical breast pain—it comes in cycles and is related to menstruation and it is caused by water retention and distension of tissues during the menstrual cycle. Different parts of the breast respond differently to the tides of hormones that flood the breast each month. Small cysts swell and collapse. Sometimes pain begins at the time of ovulation (two weeks before menstruation) and lasts until the period arrives. Sometimes it comes a few days before the period. It can affect one or both breasts and occasionally extends into the armpit. The pain varies in severity from minimal to moderately severe. For most patients it is a nuisance that can be tolerated and controlled, using various mild medications. It usually disappears after the menopause. Pain related to periods tends to be worst during the teens and just before the menopause. Cyclical breast pain has no relationship to cancer.

Non-cyclical pain refers to a localized tender area in the breast and has no relationship to periods. This may be due to cysts or fibrocystic change. Often no definite cause is found. In general, cancer is painless and mostly this pain has nothing to do with cancer. However, occasionally cancer can present with non-cyclical pain and should be investigated. Textbooks in the past emphasized that breast cancer was painless. However, recent surveys show that women with breast cancer sometimes have breast pain. What is not clear is whether the pain is due to the cancer or incidental from nearby fibrocystic change. A visit to a physician and possibly a mammogram is all that is usually required to set the woman's mind to rest.[4-10]

Sometimes patients have mild inflammation in the underlying ribs and they perceive this as coming from their breast. Physical examination by a physician will readily detect that the pain is originating from the chest wall behind the breast.

Nipple discharge

Writing in the World Journal of Surgery, Dr. H.P. Leis reported that nipple discharges could be classified into seven types:[11] milky, multicolored and sticky, purulent (pus), clear (watery), yellow (serous), pink (serosanguinous), and bloody or bloodstained.

Only the last four needed surgical investigation. The others were due to pregnancy or infections and the cause was obvious.

There are many causes of nipple discharge and cancer is the least likely. One of the most common causes of bloodstained nipple discharge is a duct papilloma. This is a benign tumor of duct epithelial cells and often is no more than the size of a pinhead.

Nipple discharge was the presenting symptom in 7.4 percent of 8,703 patients having breast operations. Fourteen percent were due to cancer and another seven percent were due to precancerous changes. The remainder were benign. The message here is that nipple discharges are usually benign. However, if they are clear, yellow, pink or bloodstained they need to be investigated.[12,13] If the nipple secretion has an associated lump it is more likely to be due to cancer.

Nipple soreness

Eczema, other skin rashes, or infection may cause nipple soreness. A nipple infection in someone who is breast feeding is due to bacterial contamination of cracked skin. It is often very painful but responds to antibiotics. However, a special type of cancer also causes soreness. Paget's disease of the nipple is due to cancer spreading from the underlying breast ducts into the epidermis (outer layer of skin).[14] Early on, it produces a nipple rash and soreness. If left untreated, it spreads to the areola (dark skin around the nipple), and eventually it will ulcerate and spread to the skin beside the areola. Some cancers invade the connective tissue directly beneath the nipple and pull the nipple inwards. This is nipple retraction or inversion. Nipple abnormalities are often present at birth, so it is important to distinguish between recent changes and retraction that has been present since childhood. Some benign conditions, such as duct ectasia, can also cause nipple retraction.

Skin changes away from the nipple

Cancers close to the surface of the breast, as they enlarge, may produce skin changes. The skin may become slightly thickened or dimpled. Sometimes little bumps appear in the skin or just under the skin. Another change is "peau d'orange" where the skin resembles the skin of an orange. Some carcinomas turn parts of the skin red, hot, sore and inflamed. These are termed inflammatory carcinomas.

Symptoms or signs due to metastases

Occasionally, a patient will find a lump under the arm and the breast will appear normal. A small cancer may sit hidden within the breast and spread to the lymph nodes in the armpit; the patient notices a lump in the armpit (metastasis) and is unaware of the breast lump. In this case, the primary breast tumor reveals itself only after a thorough examination or in a mammogram. There are many causes of benign lumps in the armpit and these must be distinguished from metastatic cancer. Rarely, metastatic cancer presents with metastases to distant organs. These can cause anything from bone pain or fractures to epilepsy or stroke.

The Decision

The family doctor

When the doctor has taken the case history and examined the breasts and the armpits, he or she then has to form an opinion about the likely significance of symptoms and signs (what the examination revealed).

There are a number of possibilities:

- There is no evidence of any abnormality
- There is a minor abnormality with a high probability that it is benign and of no consequence
- There is an abnormality that is probably benign, but the doctor has some doubt that it might be malignant
- There is an abnormality and the doctor is equally divided about the probability of benign vs. malignant
- The abnormality is suspicious for malignancy
- The doctor is certain (as it is possible to be, on clinical grounds) that it is malignant.

Based on the clinical findings, the family doctor will decide on a course of action. This will usually be one of three possibilities: reassure the patient that there is no reason for concern, refer the patient for a mammogram, or refer her to a surgeon for an expert opinion and possibly biopsy.

One could argue logically that every patient should have a mammogram. After all isn't the whole idea behind mammography to find small, early cancers before they produce a lump? This logic breaks down when we consider the patient's age. Three facts make mammography unhelpful in young patients (under the age of 40). First, breast cancer is vanishingly rare in this group. Second, even if a small cancer were present it is unlikely that mammography would find it. As the chapter on screening explains, dense breast tissue makes small cancers difficult to identify in young patients. Third, abnormalities that appear suspicious for malignancy in this age group are likely to be benign and these may lead to unnecessary surgery (a false positive mammogram).

There are exceptions to everything. If a young woman has a strong family history of breast cancer it would be logical to carry out mammography for two reasons. The incidence of cancer in these patients is high and justifies the long shot of finding anything. Second, this patient is likely to participate in a lifelong screening program and mammograms give a baseline for comparison with future regular mammograms.

A typical case for reassurance without further investigations would be a highly anxious woman in her twenties who comes to her doctor because she's frightened but has no symptoms. She may have seen something about early breast cancer on TV or knows someone who has just been diagnosed with this condition. In these circumstances the family doctor will correctly reassure the patient after physical examination reveals no abnormality.

In the past, doctors commonly reassured middle aged and older patients with minor abnormalities that these were benign. They usually told them to return in six months to confirm that no significant change had taken place. Today, in similar circumstances, most doctors would advise a mammogram and delay the final decision until they have the results.

The surgeon, the radiologist, the pathologist, and the biopsy

If the family doctor is suspicious of malignancy, or has a suspicious mammography report, or finds a lump about which he is unsure, he refers the patient to a surgeon. To speed up the process he will probably order a mammogram, with a copy of the result to go directly to the surgeon. When the surgeon sees the patient for the first time he will have the family doctor's and the radiologist's reports. Based on these reports and a clinical examination, the surgeon then has a number of options: reassure the patient that everything is okay, order further investigations, or explain to the patient that she needs some form of biopsy and go ahead with it.

The second option above might include repeat or magnified mammography views or ultrasound examination, depending on what the radiologist found. The surgeon has two office procedures of value, either a fine needle aspiration or needle core biopsy (Figure 7.2). The choice of procedure depends on a number of variables, which include the nature and size of the lump, the personal preferences of the surgeon, and the pathology services available. While the idea of fine needle aspiration is very attractive to some surgeons, others find it unreliable. It is quick, cost-effective, almost painless, and has a high degree of specificity. However, it needs great skill in obtaining a good quality specimen and it requires specially trained pathologists to interpret the findings. It is less sensitive than core biopsy. This means that any abnormality that is present (benign or malignant) is more likely to be detected by core biopsy. The core biopsy has fewer false negatives. With modern instruments, core biopsy is no more uncomfortable than fine needle aspiration. Whichever procedure opted for, the surgeon is likely to need four or more samples to ensure that the abnormality is sampled adequately.

If there is no palpable abnormality in the breast but something suspicious appears in the mammogram, this requires some form of radiology controlled biopsy. The radiologist, armed with super-sophisticated computerized imaging equipment, can guide a needle into the heart of the abnormality and take numerous small biopsies. The widespread use of

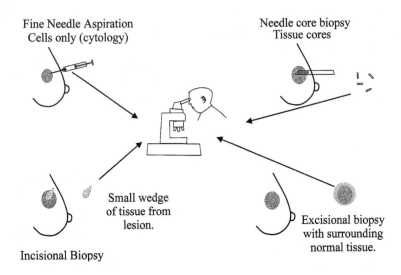

Fine Needle Aspiration
Cells only (cytology)

Needle core biopsy
Tissue cores

Small wedge
of tissue from
lesion.

Incisional Biopsy

Excisional biopsy
with surrounding
normal tissue.

Figure 7.2. Types of Biopsy

mammography has led to many more biopsies than in the past. The increased biopsy rate has spawned new ingenious tools for getting cells and tissue. There are numerous instruments on the market. Newer instruments allow radiologists to take up to ten cores, or even more, if necessary, through one small skin incision. However, four or five cores are usually adequate. Some of the new instruments allow surgeons to remove entire small tumors with the "biopsy" instrument.

As radiologists and surgeons gained experience with smaller and subtler mammographic abnormalities they have refined their choices, depending on their own experience and the experience of the medical "team" involved in the management of patients with breast disease. In some institutions, a pathologist with special training in cytopathology carries out the FNA on all symptomatic breast lumps. The same pathologist examines the cells under the microscope. These pathologists claim a much higher degree of sensitivity and accuracy than surgeons.

In many institutions, surgeons and radiologists have, for practical purposes, abandoned the use of breast fine needle aspiration and have gone over completely to the core biopsy technique. Some institutions and individuals continue to use FNA; they find it simpler, quicker, and just as useful. So, how the final diagnosis is reached depends often on local circumstances, experience, and facilities.

The chapter on screening mentioned the triple assessment conference. Difficult cases are discussed here. A typical scenario would run something like this. The woman has no symptoms and no lump. The abnormality on the mammogram is difficult to interpret but probably benign. Should we accept that it is and wait for a follow-up mammogram in one or two years? Or should we biopsy now and confirm that it is benign? There is no correct answer. Previous experience, the statistical chance of benign vs. malignant in a particular context, and what the medical literature has to say in such circumstances, will influence the decision. Ultimately, after the situation and options have been explained to the woman, she may have to make the decision. In general, if it is an early cancer, a few months' delay is unlikely to jeopardize the chance of a cure. However, for many women, a few months of uncertainty is too long and they will opt for biopsy.

Another less common situation arises when a clinically suspicious lump has an equally suspicious mammogram, but the FNA is negative. The decision here is easy. The patient needs a biopsy. The pathologist will review the biopsy to try to find the reason for the discrepancy between the mammogram and the microscopic appearance. It may be that the needle aspirate did not sample malignant cells. This is a sampling error. Sampling error is less likely with a core biopsy. If an experienced surgeon is confident that the lump is cancer clinically, and an experienced radiologist says that the mammogram is malignant, why not just go ahead and treat as cancer? There is a good reason for insisting on a positive tissue diagnosis before proceeding with treatment. It is never possible to be 100 percent sure on clinical or radiological grounds. Sometimes, conditions such as sclerosing adenosis or duct ectasia resemble cancer to such an extent that they can fool experienced radiologists and surgeons. These conditions require biopsy for confirmation but do not require wide excision. Treatment, based on clinical or mammographic appearances, might mean mastectomy. Clearly, this is undesirable and unjustified. In my experience, mastectomy is never performed without biopsy confirmation of malignancy. However, in the past, this was not always the case.

What if the core biopsy is negative and the surgeon and radiologist are convinced the lesion is malignant? It is obvious that another biopsy is necessary, and the question now is what type of biopsy. If the original was a core biopsy, they could just do a repeat core biopsy, but sometimes it might be better to move on to a larger biopsy. This means an incision or excision biopsy, and would be carried out under general anesthetic (Figure 7.2). Once this has been agreed, another option becomes available. It is possible to get a "frozen section" diagnosis during surgery. This is a form of rapid pathologic diagnosis. The surgeon removes a piece of tumor (about 1 cm) and the pathologist prepares a microscopic section for immediate diagnosis (immediate means about 15 to 20 minutes). In the past, frozen section diagnosis was very commonly performed. In general, it is not suitable for DCIS and is reserved for abnormalities producing a lump, where a non-operative diagnosis was not possible.

Before mammography, FNA, and needle biopsy became available, frozen sections were used much more commonly. The surgeon went to the operating room with a clinical diagnosis only. The treatment options were mastectomy or no mastectomy and frozen section diagnosis solved the problem during surgery. Now, the surgeon goes to the operating room with a preoperative tissue diagnosis and has a number of different options. Most of these focus on removing the tumor and leaving behind as much normal breast as possible. However, mastectomy, for some women, is still the best treatment.

Any prolonged difficulty in getting a definitive diagnosis, as discussed above, is exceptionally unusual. Most cancers are diagnosed with the first biopsy.

Treatment

After the diagnosis comes treatment. Optimal treatment varies from patient to patient, and depends on many factors. These include:

- Type—whether it is in situ or invasive
- Size of the tumor
- Stage—whether it is confined to the breast or has spread to lymph nodes or to distant organs
- Patient's general health
- Patient's age
- Patient's preference.

Almost all patients have some form of surgery. Many patients benefit from additional chemotherapy or radiotherapy either alone or in combination.[1] Some patients also opt for some form of alternative or complementary medicine (often unknown to their doctors).

Surgery

In the past, neither patient nor doctor gave much consideration to therapeutic options. A diagnosis of cancer meant mastectomy, sometimes followed by radiotherapy. The surgeon decided the type of mastectomy. This decision, as to what was the best treatment, was based on textbook dogma. This in turn reflected the personal opinion of the author and often was not based on sound, proven principles.

Many surgeons believed that William Halsted's operation, dating back to 1890, was best. In this operation, the surgeon removes the entire breast with the underlying pectoral muscles and all the lymph nodes in the axilla (armpit). This is a radical mastectomy. The pectoral muscles sit in front of the rib cage and attach themselves to the shoulder. They help control arm movements. Halsted believed that it was logical and best to remove as much tissue surrounding the breast as was surgically possible, and many of his patients did well after this operation. He felt this success vindicated his operation and until the late 1970s this mutilating procedure had a large surgical following. There was no proof that Halsted was wrong. However, there was an equal lack of proof that he was right. Not all surgeons carried out the Halsted operation. Others used a less radical procedure called a "modified" radical mastectomy. Usually they removed less muscle and performed a low axillary dissection rather than a complete axillary clearance. Some surgeons removed the breast only (no muscle). This is a simple mastectomy. Often they sampled the axillary nodes also, but did not do a major axillary dissection.

In 1985, a multicenter trial proved that mastectomy is unnecessary for most patients. Lumpectomy followed by radiotherapy gives results that are just as good.[2] The results of this and many other trials changed surgical opinion and exploded the Halsted myth.[1,3-5] We now know that the type of operation makes no difference to survival. The type of surgery does not decide whether the patient will live or die. As everyone expected, local recurrence rates were higher in the breast-conserving group—approximately ten percent. Local recurrence after mastectomy is approximately five percent. Most studies show that local recurrence after breast-conserving surgery does not affect survival, although recent studies claim that older studies are inaccurate and that it does adversely affect long-term outcome.[6]

Since the 1970s, something else has influenced surgical practice: The incidence of DCIS has increased. In the past, ductal carcinoma in situ accounted for only one to five percent of breast cancers. In 1998, in the U.S., the incidence was 17 percent. This increase is due largely to early detection by widespread use of mammography.

Surgeons treated DCIS by radical or simple mastectomy. This was because they believed that DCIS involved the entire duct system within the breast. We now know that this is not true. DCIS usually affects only one breast segment (figure 4.4). Until recently neither surgeons nor pathologists were concerned with the niceties of tumor classification. Once they knew the diagnosis was DCIS, mastectomy followed automatically. Pathologists and surgeons (and radiotherapists) no longer confine their interests to the diagnosis. They subclassify and grade DCIS (sometimes confusingly). Clinical studies confirm that classification and grade, along with the width of the surgical margins, influence recurrence rates.[78] Importantly, they now know that DCIS is completely curable in almost every patient, and usually without losing a breast. A high proportion of women now have breast-conserving surgery.

The rationale for surgery is simple. Remove the entire tumor—leave nothing behind. Mastectomy ensures that the entire tumor is removed, locally. What it cannot do is remove cells that have spread outside the breast. Advocates of radical mastectomy thought that by removing the underlying muscle and the draining lymph nodes they would guarantee complete removal. Unfortunately, this is not the case. The facts show that the type of surgery does not prolong survival.

Surgical excision less than a mastectomy strives to combine the same chance for cure, with preservation of the breast. This is breast-conserving surgery. The idea is to remove the entire tumor and a rim or margin of surrounding normal breast tissue. Surgeons call this a "lumpectomy" (Figure 8.1). Some tumors are not suitable for breast-conserving surgery. Various forms of breast reconstruction are possible after the initial surgery. Reconstructive surgery and good breast prostheses can give the woman a satisfactory cosmetic result.

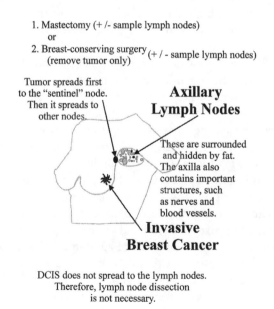

1. Mastectomy (+ /- sample lymph nodes)
   or
2. Breast-conserving surgery (+ / - sample lymph nodes)
   (remove tumor only)

Tumor spreads first to the "sentinel" node. Then it spreads to other nodes.

Axillary Lymph Nodes

These are surrounded and hidden by fat. The axilla also contains important structures, such as nerves and blood vessels.

Invasive Breast Cancer

DCIS does not spread to the lymph nodes. Therefore, lymph node dissection is not necessary.

Figure 8.1. Surgery for Breast Cancer

Until relatively recently, surgeons often dissected axillary lymph nodes when they were removing DCIS. As we might have anticipated, they found no tumor in the axilla. However, it took a clinical trial to show that axillary dissection was an unnecessary procedure for patients with DCIS. Axillary dissection is no longer performed in DCIS patients, except in the unusual situation where it is extensive and requires a mastectomy. Extensive DCIS may contain a few hidden foci of invasive cancer with metastatic potential.

How does a surgeon decide whether breast-conserving surgery or mastectomy is most appropriate? The National Cancer Institute offers guidelines. Breast-conserving surgery is suitable for DCIS and for most invasive cancers if they can be excised with a rim of normal breast tissue, i.e., with surgical margins free of tumor cells. Up to 80 percent of breast cancers are suitable for breast-conserving surgery. Mastectomy is usually the best choice for women with a large tumor, or with small breasts, or with multiple tumors in different parts of the breast. It is usually the best choice for tumors involving many ducts directly beneath the nipple. It may also be the surgical treatment of choice for patients whose cancers are discovered during early pregnancy.[9] In these circumstances it is difficult to achieve a good cosmetic result with breast-conserving surgery, and local recurrence rates are high. An aggressive tumor or the presence of metastases does not contraindicate breast-conserving surgery. Nor does the patient's age.

In 1991, the National Cancer Institute, a branch of the National Institutes of Health, urged surgeons and hospitals to move from mastectomy to lumpectomy. Many doctors paid little heed to this advice.[10-13] In the mid–1990s only 20 percent of patients considered suitable for mastectomy were benefiting from this operation. Why were the other 80 percent still having mastectomies? Even as we enter the new century surgeons are still performing too many mastectomies. Why?

There are many possible explanations, mostly to do with doctors' attitudes. Some older surgeons, trained to perform mastectomies, are reluctant to switch to the technically more demanding surgery. It is more difficult to remove part of a breast and produce a good cosmetic result than to remove an entire breast. Some surgeons admit they don't trust the results of the clinical trials. Some say they don't know the long-term consequences of radiation, despite the evidence gathered over decades indicating that breast radiotherapy is safe. But what about the organs behind the breast? In the past, long-term complications of breast radiation included damage to the coronary arteries and lungs lying in the chest behind the left breast. Newer radiation techniques avoid damage to the heart and lungs.[14]

Surgeons report that patients frequently insist on mastectomies. Some women feel that mastectomy is a more comprehensive treatment, and they do not want radiotherapy or the risk of local recurrence. Critics of surgeons who do not perform lumpectomies have other views. They say surgeons don't want to hand over breast cancer leadership to other specialists—radiotherapists and medical oncologists. They also accuse surgeons of giving information to patients in a way that prejudices them in favor of mastectomy. They accuse surgeons of taking the attitude that older women don't need their breasts. Breast cancer is most common in older women. If a surgeon tells a patient his or her preference is mastectomy, the patient usually goes along with this. The type of hospital also seems to influence the choice of surgery offered to women. If you check which hospitals have the highest incidence of mastectomy, you will find that, in general, these are smaller hospitals. Large cancer centers and university hospitals treat most patients by lumpectomy.

Another factor that influences the choice of surgery is patient preference. Many women, understandably, have a strong wish to keep both breasts. Some do not, and feel more comfortable knowing that not only is the tumor removed but also that the breast that was home for this cancer is also gone. Other factors influencing the patients' choice include media coverage and the treatment given to women in high places, be they politicians, film stars, or the wives of such famous people.

Shortly after Nancy Reagan had a modified radical mastectomy in 1987, the rates for breast-conserving surgery dropped off and doctors attributed the drop-off to media coverage.[15,16] This decrease was in middle-aged and older women, age 50–79 years (most patients are in this age range), and was most apparent among white women. There were geographical regional differences also.[10,11,13,17] As the publicity died down, women started to opt again for conserving surgery and this trend was most apparent in women with a higher educational background.

Population statistics show that in the U.S., in 1983, the rate for breast-conserving surgery was 14 percent. This had risen to 35 percent in 1990. By 1994, the figure was 44 percent for patients with early breast cancer. If surgical guidelines were adhered to, this figure should be approximately 80 percent. The statistics also show that surgeons are less likely to perform conserving surgery in patients over 60.

Overall, breast experts are disappointed with the low rate of breast-conserving surgery. They are also concerned that less than 80 percent of these patients receive postoperative radiation therapy. Regional figures show that in the Eastern U.S. 58 percent of women receive conserving surgery, compared to 48 percent on the West Coast and 33 percent in the

South. Ethnic minorities also appear to have fewer breast-conserving procedures than white women.[18] Numerous studies confirm that there is great variation in the treatment offered to women.

Mastectomy patients opting for breast reconstruction can have it done at the same time as mastectomy, or as a separate operation at a later date. The type of reconstruction depends on a number of medical variables and on the patient's choice. Most patients will choose some form of silicone or saline implant. Others will prefer reconstruction from their own tissue taken from the abdomen or back.

Reconstruction usually occurs in stages. In the first stage the surgeon restores the general size and shape of the breast. The second stage restores breast symmetry, nipple, and areola. The cosmetic outcome after breast-conserving surgery depends on such factors as the surgeon's experience, the size of the tumor, the size of the breast, the extent of surgery required, and the response of the patient to radiation treatment. On a four-point scale (excellent, good, fair or poor) 80 to 90 percent of patients get an excellent or good result. Oncolink, the web site at the University of Pennsylvania cancer center, has excellent information on breast reconstruction surgery. It also contains a list of frequently asked questions about reconstruction. It can be found at http://www.oncolink.upenn.edu/disease/breast/treat/recon/.

Should lymph nodes be removed? Yes, sometimes. Pathological examination of the cancer and a few lymph nodes gives useful information about the aggressiveness of the tumor. It also gives some idea whether the tumor is likely to have spread beyond the breast and axilla. This pathology information acts as a pointer and often determines which patients are likely to benefit from chemotherapy. Experts advise surgeons to sample about five lymph nodes in all patients with invasive breast cancer. This recommendation may change as we learn more about the biology of cancers and their responsiveness to different chemotherapy protocols. Soon, biopsy of just one lymph node, called the sentinel node (Figure 8.1), may give the medical oncologists all the information they need about whether chemotherapy is likely to benefit the patient.[19,20]

Radiation Therapy

The second treatment limb is radiotherapy. Like surgery, it is a form of local treatment. It treats the tumor bed (where the tumor was removed) and the surrounding tissue. Sometimes it also treats the axilla. X-rays kill tumor cells. They also destroy normal cells and can cause serious complications, if delivered incorrectly.

The same amount of radiation affects different cells in different ways. Some normal cells are highly resistant to radiation; others are exquisitely sensitive. So too are many tumors. In general, stable non-dividing normal cells (such as muscle cells) are radioresistant, i.e., not easily damaged, whereas rapidly dividing cells (such as bone marrow cells) are radiosensitive. Some tumors, such as certain sarcomas, are highly radioresistant whereas malignant lymphomas often melt like magic. Most malignancies lie somewhere between these extremes.

The therapeutic trick is to deliver x-rays in a way that kills tumor cells but leaves normal cells unharmed. Small (sublethal) doses cause minor damage to normal cells. However, normal cells, with intact DNA repair mechanisms, repair themselves quickly. Tumor cells lacking these normal repair mechanisms do not repair themselves well. Treatment given in multiple small fractions allows normal cells to return to normal in the interval between each treatment. Before tumor cells have time to recover a second treatment intensifies the damage caused by the first dose of rays. In this way, radiation damage to tumor cells is cumulative and lethal, whereas normal cells survive.

The effectiveness of radiotherapy first became evident in the late 1800s. Its popularity waxed and waned in the 20th century as doctors became aware of its dangers and at times its apparent lack of effectiveness, and then rediscovered its value, and discovered new safer technology. Since the 1940s, doctors knew that radiation therapy reduced local recurrence after mastectomy.

Detailed statistical analysis in the 1980s showed that although the radiotherapy reduced local recurrences, it did not reduce overall mortality. Because it did not alter mortality rates, and because there was a heightened awareness of its dangers, its routine use declined. Curiously, many patients having radiotherapy were dying earlier than expected, but not from breast cancer. If they were not dying from cancer, what was killing them?

They were dying from heart failure. It turns out that radiation was passing through the chest wall and hitting the heart (this is not surprising). The heart consists of muscle, which is radioresistant, and this was not directly damaged. However, the beams also hit the coronary arteries and produced an accelerated form of atherosclerosis (blocking of the arteries).[21,22] The risk for fatal myocardial infarction (heart attack) ten to 15 years after radiotherapy is higher for those patients who had left-sided breast radiation rather than right-sided radiation. The heart lies behind, and slightly inside the left breast. The radiation was constricting the coronary arteries and squeezing out the blood supply to the heart muscle. This in turn led to heart failure.

The realization that radiation therapy could damage the heart and reduce overall survival prevented widespread use of radiotherapy, except in very well defined circumstances. The circumstances are still being studied for optimal selection and benefit.

Modern computer-driven x-ray machines pinpoint their targets accurately. They ensure minimal damage to surrounding tissues. Radiation therapists, like their colleagues in other medical specialties, continually research new techniques that might improve treatment. Gradually, they are finding better ways to kill tumors and protect normal cells. For example, a number of medical centers are studying the technique called brachytherapy. Rather than project beams from an external source, brachytherapy uses radiation from small temporary implants within the breast. Advocates of brachytherapy claim that treatment time is shorter and there are fewer complications. However, it is not clear yet if their results are as good as those obtained by conventional radiation therapy.

Complications from radiation therapy are far less common now than in the past. We rarely see radiation burns to the skin or painful necrosis of the ribs behind the breast. Nevertheless, complications still occur. Sometimes the radiated normal breast tissue becomes firm or hard. This may be uncomfortable. It may also hinder detection of early tumor recurrence. Long-term complications, such as sarcomas in the radiated tissue, are exceptionally rare. Despite the rarity of these complications, radiotherapists are not complacent. Much of their clinical research is directed at getting the correct balance between good therapeutic effect and as few complications as possible. One of the reasons why doctors try to characterize each tumor is because individual tumors respond differently to different treatment protocols. For example, some doctors feel that radiation treatment for DCIS can be finessed, taking into account accurate tumor grading and classification. They feel that radiation treatment for all DCIS patients after breast-conserving surgery is perhaps blunderbuss treatment. They argue that patients with small tumors and negative surgical margins are unlikely to benefit from radiotherapy. They argue that there are small subgroups for whom radiation therapy is not beneficial. This is especially true for patients with low-grade ductal carcinoma in situ (DCIS).[23] Not everybody agrees.

X-rays are normally delivered from an external "gun." This directs the beam to a precisely defined area. The total dose is divided into 25 to

30 daily fractions (five days a week). The tumor size, whether or not a breast-conserving procedure was performed, and whether or not the axilla should be included all determine the localization and dose required. If reconstructive surgery is planned, this too must be taken into consideration. Numerous clinical trials show that radiotherapy is effective in destroying small numbers of cells left behind after surgery. Even in patients who have mastectomy and chemotherapy, radiotherapy reduces local recurrence and benefits long-term survival.

Ongoing trials strive to define subgroups of patients that will benefit most. In these subgroups, scientists examine different variables, such as the size of the original tumor, the closeness of the surgical margins, and the presence or absence of axillary metastases. Basic cancer research and the results of clinical trials often determine the direction of future practice. For example, it is now standard practice to include radiation treatment after breast-conserving surgery (note the reservations mentioned above). Long-term follow-up shows that such radiation treatment benefits women with cancers 4 cm or less, even if they have positive lymph nodes.

The National Cancer Institute has radiotherapy information for patients at http://cancernet.nci.nih.gov/clinpdq/therapy/Radiotherapy.html.[24]

There is also excellent information at http://www.medsch.wisc.edu/bca/faq/radiation.html.[25,26]

We now know from large Canadian and Danish studies published in the New England Journal of Medicine, in 1997, that the combination of radiation therapy and chemotherapy is more effective than chemotherapy alone in achieving long-term survival. Dr. Joseph Ragaz, in a major study from Vancouver, found that combined chemotherapy and radiotherapy reduced mortality by 30 percent, in comparison to chemotherapy alone. This was after 15 years of follow-up, and in women with lymph node metastases.[27] Meanwhile, colleagues across the Atlantic in Denmark found similar results,[28] and published these in the same issue of the journal.

At least, we know that this is true for high-risk premenopausal women who have had mastectomy. Oncologists hope that the same results will apply to other patients who receive radiation therapy after conservative surgery.

Chemotherapy

Before the 1970s, the specialty of medical oncology as we know it today did not exist. Surgeons and radiotherapists treated cancer patients.

Now, medical oncologists contribute significantly to the management of breast cancer patients, and their main tool is chemotherapy. Chemotherapy is a dreaded word, almost as dreaded as the word cancer. It conjures up images of baldness, paleness, and vomiting. However, in recent years new drugs are highly effective in preventing many of the side effects. In particular, for most patients, the horrendous nausea of previous decades has gone. Pallor is mostly due to anemia and if necessary this can be treated safely with blood transfusions. Soon, new marrow-stimulating drugs may reduce the need for blood transfusions. Excellent wigs, to some extent, counteract the potential feeding of nakedness and self-consciousness that comes with total hair loss. New drugs are highly effective in treating life-threatening infections (a major problem in the past). Still, no matter what way you package the news about advances in cancer care, chemotherapy is tough.

Previously, chemotherapy was reserved for exceptionally high-risk patients—those with distant metastases. This was palliative treatment. Although it often added a few months to the patient's survival it rarely cured anyone. It was too toxic to give to low risk patients. Its benefit was not obvious and the attitude of most doctors was that it did more harm than good. Its use was rarely justified. As better drugs became available, and as side effects became preventable or minimized, clinical trials tested the value of chemotherapy in earlier stage disease. Firstly, they showed that it was valuable in patients with lymph node metastases, and later its value was proven for some patients with no identifiable metastases. Patients with large primary tumors, or with aggressive (high grade) primary tumors of any size, are at risk for metastases, even if none are found at the time of surgery. The trend is to use chemotherapy at a much earlier stage than previously.

Chemotherapy works differently from surgery and radiotherapy. The surgeon removes visible tumor, with a "safe" margin of surrounding tissue. This margin may be a rim of normal breast tissue or the entire breast. However, the surgeon has no way of knowing if tumor cells have strayed beyond this margin. Likewise even if the surgeon removes axillary lymph nodes there may still be stray tumor cells hiding somewhere in the armpit. Imagine a large weed sitting in a lawn with its roots spreading out below ground level. The gardener digs the ground around the weed and its roots. If he is lucky, all the roots will come easily and intact. This is what the surgeon does. Some of the root' s tips may remain behind. The gardener can spray weed killer on the surrounding earth and kill the hidden roots. This is what the radiotherapist does. He also sprays x-rays into the axilla in the hope of killing any tiny metastases. Most breast cancers are sensitive to radiation and are killed by the x-rays. Some are resistant, and these grow again at a later stage. They are responsible for local recurrences.

Surgery and radiotherapy are forms of "local" treatment. Chemotherapy is systemic treatment. Just as we use antibiotics to kill bugs hidden in the nooks and crannies of our lungs or elsewhere, we use chemotherapy to seek and destroy tumor cells that have traveled beyond the surgical and radiation fields. Unfortunately, these chemical missiles are not smart enough to know the difference between friend and foe. They damage normal cells as well as tumor cells. Someone once described chemotherapy as like throwing a bomb and hoping that it would kill more enemies than friends. Newer drugs and delivery methods limit the damage. Doctors deliver these agents of death and destruction (for tumor cells) in different sequences, so that they can target every part of the cell cycle. However, they still inflict considerable damage on the normal cell population.

Unlike normal cells, tumor cells spend different time periods in the various phases of their cell cycle (Figure 8.2). They stop and start unpredictably. Different chemicals and enzymes control different phases of the cell cycle. At any one time, groups of tumor cells are in different parts of the cycle.

To use a science-fiction war analogy—imagine a building with the alien enemy controlling vital machines (e.g., computers). They have human hostages. Your task is to destroy the enemy without demolishing the building (the body) or the hostages.

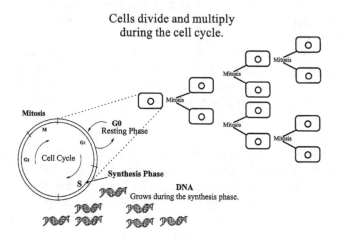

Figure 8.2. Cell Cycle

With various chemotherapy combinations, oncologists can kill the enemy. However, killing the enemy is only half the problem. Their drugs also destroy normal cells, and these must be preserved if the patient is to survive. In general, chemotherapy works best on cells that are dividing rapidly and hardly touches cells that lie dormant and inactive.

As mentioned above, normal cells fit into three main categories with regard to their ability to divide. For convenience, we call these rapidly dividing, slowly dividing, and non-dividing cells. Those that divide frequently, such as bone marrow, intestine, and hair follicle cells are hit most by chemotherapy. Bone marrow makes white blood cells to fight infection, red blood cells to carry oxygen (bound to hemoglobin), and platelets to stop bleeding after minor injury. White cells are the most sensitive to chemotherapy. Chemotherapy is lethal to tumor cells but in high doses it wipes out normal bone marrow. Oncologists monitor marrow function by examining the patients' white blood cells. As marrow function decreases the white cell count drops. New drugs stimulate the marrow and can raise the white cell count when necessary. GCSF (granulocyte colony stimulating factor) is an amazing new drug. It specifically instructs marrow white cells to grow and divide, without significantly affecting other cells. It saves lives by giving back to the body its ability to fight infections, infections that would be trivial for the normal person but fatal for patients without their protective white cells. Other drugs can also specifically stimulate platelets and red blood cells and are useful for other medical disorders, but are not yet so useful for cancer patients. When cancer patients need platelets or red cells, doctors give them blood transfusions. These tide the patient over the short-term crises that arise periodically during chemotherapy.

Single drugs are not as effective as multiple drugs because they hit only one part of the cell cycle. Most tumor cells are not synchronized—different cells are in different cycles. Using drug combinations, the oncologist tries to hit all tumor cells, regardless of what part of the cell cycle they occupy. One major obstacle is the resting phase (called the G0 phase). During this phase cells are resistant to drugs, and at any one time many or most tumor cells are in the resting phase. So, even if you could poison all dividing tumor cells using a heavy dose of combined chemotherapy the bulk of the tumor would survive. The total number of tumor cells (tumor cell burden) is an important factor limiting the effectiveness of chemotherapy. Most cancers are at least 1 cm before they are detected. A 1 cm tumor contains approximately 10^9 cells, at diagnosis, and many tumors have more than 10^{10} cancer cells (10 billion cells, or approximately 10 grams of tumor).

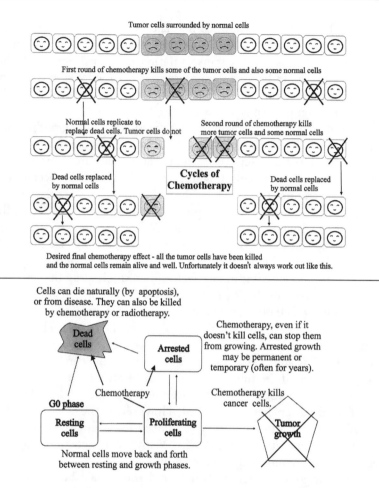

Tumor cells surrounded by normal cells

First round of chemotherapy kills some of the tumor cells and also some normal cells

Normal cells replicate to replace dead cells. Tumor cells do not

Second round of chemotherapy kills more tumor cells and some normal cells

Dead cells replaced by normal cells

Cycles of Chemotherapy

Dead cells replaced by normal cells

Desired final chemotherapy effect - all the tumor cells have been killed and the normal cells remain alive and well. Unfortunately it doesn't always work out like this.

Cells can die naturally (by apoptosis), or from disease. They can also be killed by chemotherapy or radiotherapy.

Dead cells

Arrested cells

Chemotherapy, even if it doesn't kill cells, can stop them from growing. Arrested growth may be permanent or temporary (often for years).

G0 phase

Chemotherapy

Resting cells

Proliferating cells

Chemotherapy kills cancer cells.

Tumor growth

Normal cells move back and forth between resting and growth phases.

Figure 8.3 (top) *Cycles of Chemotherapy and*
Figure 8.4 (bottom) *Chemotheraphy Hits Dividing Cells*

Theoretically, even if the drug killed 99.99 percent of the tumor cells, 1 to 10 million cells would remain. If the tumor is chemosensitive, the repeated cycles will destroy the remainder of the tumor cells after they leave the resting phase. Chemotherapy is a prolonged process. It is given over a period of days or weeks and then repeated many times. The total duration may be many months. During the intervals between doses, normal cells get a chance to recover, and resting tumor cells move into a susceptible phase of the cycle. The next course of chemotherapy will kill some of these (Figure 8.3). Hopefully, even if a few tumor cells remain alive, they will remain dormant for the remainder of the patient's life (Figure 8.4). Chemotherapy is likely to be most successful when the cancer cell population is small and the likelihood of large numbers of resistant or metastatic cells is remote. Recent hopes that stem cell transplantation combined with high dose chemotherapy would be a new way forward for patients with metastatic breast cancer have not been fulfilled. Current trial results show that chemotherapy on its own is just as good.[29,30]

A second major factor influencing the success of chemotherapy is drug resistance. Even if a tiny number of tumor cells are drug-resistant these may re-grow in a few years. Some tumor cells are resistant to all forms of chemotherapy (multidrug resistance). They contain specific genes that produce an unusual protein on the cell surface. This is called P–glycoprotein and its function is to prevent certain chemicals (including chemotherapy drugs) from entering the cell. Furthermore, if chemotherapy drugs succeed in entering, the glycoprotein rapidly ejects them.[31-33]

Combination chemotherapy is used for most patients requiring chemotherapy, because it is more effective than single-drug therapy. How do we know this? Oncologists have studied different drug regimes in 400 trials, involving 220,000 women, over the past 25 years. Their recommendations are based on meticulous analyses of the results. The benefits are most obvious in younger women, especially those who are premenopausal. The addition of Tamoxifen reduces local recurrence rates and prolongs survival, if the tumor cells are positive for estrogen receptors.

Some women discover breast cancer during pregnancy and the question of termination has to be faced. However, if the woman wishes, chemotherapy can often be safely postponed for a few weeks, until the fetus has developed to a viable stage.[34] Many women come through the pregnancy and chemotherapy successfully.

Some drugs are taken as tablets and some must be given intravenously. They are tailored to the individual patient's requirements to maximize their toxic effect on different phases of the cell cycle and at the same time to inflict minimal damage on normal cells.

While the side effects and complications of chemotherapy have diminished considerably in recent years, they have not disappeared. Doctors now have better remedies to counteract and minimize side effects. The discovery of the drug GCSF has dramatically reduced infections resulting from chemotherapy. This, in turn, has reduced the mortality from serious infections, the need for antibiotics, the side effects of antibiotics, and the overall need for patients to remain in hospital for long periods of time. Better antibiotics stamp out infections. The antifungal drugs quickly dispel the soreness that accompanies fungal mouth and skin infections (called thrush or candida). Systemic (e.g., lung and other deep tissues) viral infections are less life threatening than in the past. However, they can still be fatal. New anti-sickness (antiemetic) drugs have almost abolished the relentless and demoralizing nausea and vomiting that accompanied chemotherapy in the past. For many patients, the sickness after chemotherapy, if it is present at all, is little more than a mild hangover. Some patients have vague non-specific symptoms that are difficult to counteract. Common side effects are fatigue and tiredness. Often patients find that they feel listless and sleep a lot.

Sometimes chemotherapy causes long-term complications. Peripheral neuropathy is a form of damage to nerve endings. Nerve damage causes tingling and loss of sensation in the fingers and feet. Often it is mild and transient, and gets better when chemotherapy is stopped. Sometimes the neuropathy is permanent. Some drugs if given in high dose may cause heart failure. Some drugs are more likely to produce side effects than others and the susceptibility to complications varies from patient to patient.

Young women may become infertile. Sometimes fertility cannot be restored. Exciting new research holds out the possibility of removing ova before chemotherapy and transplanting them after chemotherapy, to restore fertility (Source: ReutersHealth, Jan. 2000). Many women go through an early menopause. Hormone replacement treatment can alleviate symptoms. The following website gives a good overview of cancer therapy and how it affects fertility[35]: http://www.cancernews.com/articles/cancer&fertility.htm.

One potential long-term complication is the development of a new cancer. Years after chemotherapy is finished, a minuscule number of patients get a second cancer unrelated to the breast cancer. Often this is leukemia. We use cytotoxic chemotherapy to kill cancer cells. However, these are also mutagens. They damage DNA. Rarely these mutations cause new malignancies. This usually happens three to five years later. The National Cancer Institute has chemotherapy information for patients at its website,[36] cancernet.nci.nih.gov/peb/chemo_you/.

Hormone Treatment

Estrogen appears to be an important hormone in promoting breast cancer growth. Many tumors contain estrogen receptors on the surface of the tumor cells. These receptors bind to estrogen, which in turn stimulates cell growth. There are a number of ways to block this effect. In the past, surgeons commonly removed the patients' ovaries, thus reducing the amount of circulating estrogen. They often achieved the same effect by radiating the ovaries. Today, they can do the same thing with drugs.

Tamoxifen is the most widely prescribed anti–breast cancer drug. This works by blocking the estrogen receptors from binding to estrogen. This prevents the estrogen from acting on the tumor cells. For many years oncologists have known the benefit of Tamoxifen in reducing symptoms in advanced breast cancer. It produces similar effects to ovarian ablation. They wondered if it might be beneficial also in early breast cancer. It is. Fifty-five clinical trials have studied 37,000 women with stage one and two breast cancer, and their findings confirm that Tamoxifen is beneficial in reducing local recurrence and mortality.[37] It is beneficial in all age groups if the tumor cells are estrogen receptor-positive. As we might expect, it is not effective for patients whose tumors are estrogen receptor-negative. Doctors usually prescribe Tamoxifen for five years. Treatment for longer than this does not appear to add any additional benefit. It has relatively few side effects and is inexpensive. However, it is associated with a slight increase in cancer of the uterus. This uterine cancer is usually low-grade, easily treated, and rarely fatal. Recent information from epidemiologists suggest that Tamoxifen is a highly effective breast cancer drug.

Alternative Medicine

Increasingly, patients want more than conventional medicine. In 1990, 34 percent of Americans saw an alternative health care practitioner, constituting almost 400 million visits, costing an estimated $13 billion.[38] In 1997, the number of visits had increased to 630 million.

Alternative medicine is difficult to define precisely; loosely defined it refers to practices "neither taught widely in medical schools nor generally available in hospitals." However, it falls into seven main categories [39–42]: diet and nutrition, mind-body techniques, bioelectromagnetics, traditional folk remedies, pharmacologic, manual healing methods, and herbal medicine.

In the past, doctors viewed alternative medicine as synonymous with quackery, often with good reason. In 1861 an American physician writing in the National Quarterly Review said, "Quackery kills a larger number annually of the citizens of the United States than all of the disease it pretends to cure."[43] Cancer patients, in particular those with terminal disease, are vulnerable and will grasp at any hope, however slim.

Without doubt, quackery is still alive and thriving in the United States. While a small number of these alternative treatments are dangerous, most are harmless. However, as far as we know, they have no curative effect. This is where the main clash with conventional medicine occurs. Despite passionate claims from patients and many practitioners, there is no scientific evidence that alternative therapies cure cancer. Conventional medicine argues that it is inappropriate to support unproven remedies. Alternative medicine advocates claim they have not been given a fair chance to prove the value of their treatments. They argue that billions of dollars are pumped into conventional medical research while they have had no opportunity to prove their theories.

In response to public and political pressure, Congress created the Office of Alternative Medicine (OAM) in 1992 at the National Institutes of Health. In 1992, the OAM had a budget of $2 million. In 1997, this had grown to $12 million. In 1999, it is estimated that the NIH spent about $40 million on alternative medicine–related research. This is approximately 0.003 percent of its budget. The largest alternative medicine project is the shark cartilage trial. This $2.5 million research project will test the value of shark cartilage for cancer patients. Shark cartilage treatment is big business. Many scientists and non-scientists believe it is also a big fraud. Anyone looking for an insight into how the marketing of shark cartilage has been sold to the public should read Mark Jenkins' article, "The great white hype."[44] There are no reliable figures for how many people are taking shark cartilage in America. Estimates range from 25,000 to 250,000. It is considered to be a $50 million to $100 million business. Commentators estimate that one manufacturer sells more than $1 million worth each month.

The functions of the OAM are to facilitate the evaluation of alternative medical treatments, investigate and evaluate the efficacy of alternative treatments, establish an information clearinghouse to inform the public about alternative medicine, and support research training in alternative medical practices. The NCI has an alternative medicine website at http://cancernet.nci.nih.gov/treatment/cam.shtml.[45]

Despite their skepticism, doctors now accept that there are many beneficial "unconventional remedies." The term complementary medicine is often used for these treatments. Physicians will gladly support any program that helps the patient feel better, physically or psychologically. It is clear that medical students and doctors want to learn more about complementary treatments, and many medical schools have responded by offering courses. Doctors want to help their patients but do not want to waste their patients' or their own time with useless remedies. They want to protect their patients from receiving false hope and from losing a lot of cash in the process.

With regard to breast cancer, it is clear that alternative medicine has no curative effect. However, many treatments may improve a patient's well-being and play a complementary role in her road to recovery.

What type of patient seeks alternative treatments? The stereotype is portrayed as a young, middle-class, well-educated, self-assertive woman; the type of woman who wants to feel in control of her body and mind. At least that is what studies in the past have shown.[46] A recent report in the New England Journal of Medicine found something different.[47] Twenty-eight percent of 480 patients with early breast cancer sought alternative therapies after surgery. In comparison to those who did not seek such therapy, they suffered more depression, more anxiety, less sexual satisfaction, and a greater fear of recurrence. The researchers concluded, "Among women with newly diagnosed early-stage breast cancer who had been treated with standard therapies, new use of alternative medicine was a marker of greater psychosocial distress and worse quality of life."

Doctors in busy oncology clinics focus their time and effort primarily on the physical aspects of cancer. If they do not look specifically for anxiety or depression, patients may never unburden their troubles on them. Within the medical profession, it is family doctors and nurses who are showing the greatest interest in learning how to help patients in a holistic manner.

After the intense psychological trauma of the events surrounding the investigations, and diagnosis, the patient and doctor discuss which treatment is best. Doctors treat breast cancer patients in accordance with "best practice" protocols defined by their medical specialties and expert groups, and recommend these to the patient. However, every patient is slightly different and treatment must often be modified. Sometimes the modifications are necessary for specific medical reasons; at other times modifications are necessary because of a patient's wishes. Even after the doctor and patient decide on the course of treatment, it may be necessary to modify the treatment as time goes by. Sometimes patients want to be included in a clinical trial.

What Are Clinical Trials?

Clinical trials are investigations that help find the best treatment for specific diseases or problems. Before any new drug is approved for general use it must go through a testing period, first in the laboratory and then in humans. Only about one in a thousand drugs studied in the laboratory will make it to human testing. The average time for a successful laboratory test is five years. After this it goes into clinical trial; the components of a trial are called Phase I, Phase II, and Phase III.

Phase I tests the drug's safety, and investigates the best way to administer the drug. It investigates how a new drug should be administered (orally, intravenously, by injection), how often, and in what dosage. It also gathers information on how the body absorbs, metabolizes, and excretes the drug. Phase I is carried out in healthy volunteers and in a small number of patients with terminal illness usually for whom all other treatments have failed. Phase I trials last from one to three years and the study is confined to small numbers of patients (usually less than 100). Only one in five Phase I drugs makes it to the market, and this usually takes another five to nine years. Successful drugs pass to Phase II.

If the drug moves to Phase II, its chances of getting to the market improve to almost 30 percent. A Phase II trial provides preliminary information about how well the new drug works. It gathers information on possible side effects in more patients than Phase I, usually 100 to 300. This phase lasts about two years. If successful, it moves to Phase III.

Phase III tries to verify the effectiveness of the drug in large numbers of patients, often more than 1,000. Drugs that enter this phase have a 60 percent chance of getting to the market.

Phase III compares the new treatment with an existing treatment. If it is better, it will replace the old treatment. Patients are randomized. This means they do not know which treatment they are receiving. Phase III takes three to four years.

At this stage, if the trial appears beneficial, the pharmaceutical company will submit to the Food and Drug Administration what is known as a New Drug Application. This contains all the data obtained during the trial and may contain up to 100,000 pages of information. The cost of putting a drug through clinical trials is somewhere between $350 million and $500 million.

Patients often ask if they are going to be guinea pigs in some experiment. No, they are not. The rules, regulations, ethics, and criteria for carrying out clinical trials are strictly controlled. They are only carried out on patients who volunteer after getting detailed informed consent. They are conducted in accordance with internationally agreed guidelines as laid down in the Nuremberg Code (1947) and the Declaration of Helsinki (1964). Various review groups, often more than one, have to approve every study. These include the sponsoring authority (such as the National

Cancer Institute) and the Institutional Review Board (IRB) that oversees clinical research in the institution where the trial is taking place. The IRB includes doctors, other health care providers, consumers, and sometimes members of the clergy.

Patients usually go into Phase II or Phase III trials. Patients entered into Phase II trials are guaranteed they will get the new drug. The disadvantage at this stage is that the doctors have incomplete knowledge about the efficacy or side effects. Phase III trials are safer. However, patients have no guarantee they will get the new treatment. In fact, they have a 50 percent chance of getting the new one and a 50 percent chance of getting the existing treatment. Even if a patient does not receive the new treatment, she can rest assured she will be treated in the best-known way. Every aspect of her progress will be monitored carefully.

Physicians get breast cancer like everyone else, and then they become patients. They suffer the same fears and anxieties as their patients. Dr. Jane Poulson, in June 1998, touched the hearts of seasoned physicians around the world with the story of her own breast cancer and how it affected her and her attitudes. As a palliative care physician she had counseled patients with cancer for 15 years. She had given seminars on how to "break bad news" to patients. She had explained to patients the wonders of modern medical technology, how quickly the surgery was performed, and how fantastic the wigs were (after chemotherapy). Yet when it came to her own illness, she reacted with the same emotion and tears she had seen in her patients. She recalled for her medical readers her devastation at not being allowed to participate in a clinical trial for bone marrow transplantation (she did not meet the rigorous criteria required for entry).

Although patients who volunteer for clinical trials may not get the new drug, they are guaranteed the best care known to modern medicine. The doctors will meticulously monitor their progress with frequent and sophisticated testing. In general, all patients can expect to benefit in some way from participation in a clinical trial.

The NCI has a clinical trials web page at this address: http://cancertrials.nci.nih.gov/.

Prognosis: What Are the Chances of Being Cured?

When the shock of the diagnosis subsides, frightening questions flood the patient's mind. These come with varying degrees of importance and relevance. Always at the top, however, is the question "Am I going to die?"

When doctors talk about prognosis they talk about survival rates. They use phrases like two-year, five-year, and ten-year survival rates. These figures come from large studies and clinical trials and they take into account all the major risk factors associated with death. They resemble the actuarial calculations used by insurance companies to figure out whether or not an individual is a good or bad insurance risk. Another large group of "prognosticators" are weather forecasters. Their forecasting is sometimes very accurate and sometimes they get it disastrously wrong. How good they are depends to some extent on which part of the world they are forecasting for. If they say it's going to snow on the North Pole they won't be wrong very often. They also do a pretty good job when prognosticating for large landmasses such as North America. However, when it comes to predicting rain or sunshine in some parts of the world, such as the coast of Western Europe (Ireland and the United Kingdom), many locals think they could do just as well with the toss of a coin.

Doctors do not prognosticate as well as the actuaries, but do much better than many weather forecasters. Survival figures apply to groups of people with similar cancers and to subgroups of patients with similar characteristics. The statistics do not apply strictly to individual patients, but to groups of patients with the same tumor characteristics. Anyone wishing to get a better understanding of the way population statistics often do not apply to the individual should read Harvard biologist Stephen Jay Gould's brilliant essay "The Median Isn't the Message." He describes how he was diagnosed with a terrible form of cancer and how the statistics did not apply to his particular circumstances.[1] His essay is on this web site: http://www.stat.berkeley.edu/~rice/stat20_98/GouldCancer.html.

If you have breast cancer, your chance of being alive (and without disease) will be compared to a group of patients who are more or less the same age, whose tumor is the same pathologic type, and whose tumor is at the same stage of spread at the time of diagnosis. Sometimes this prognostic accuracy approaches 100 percent. More often it falls a long way short of this. This lack of accuracy is due to unforeseen variables. We never know everything about a tumor. We can measure hundreds of variables, but the tumor may hide some of its lethal weapons. These are the unknown variables. Unknown variables also prevent the insurance companies and the weather forecasters from getting it right all the time. Different variables have different prognostic strengths, and some are more reliable predictors than others. Sometimes, one or two prognostic variables make all the others irrelevant and statisticians can find these important variables using a statistical technique called multivariate analysis. What then are the variables that give the best prognostic information?

For breast cancer patients the most powerful predictor of five-year or ten-year survival (and for all practical purposes "cure") is whether the carcinoma is in situ or invasive. If the diagnosis is ductal carcinoma in situ (DCIS) the chance of complete cure approaches 100 percent. It is easy to prognosticate for DCIS regarding survival. One study of over 700 DCIS patients found that mastectomy had a cure rate of 100 percent. For those who have breast-conserving surgery and radiation treatment the recurrence rate is approximately 15 percent. Other studies have found similar results.[2,3]

In patients with breast-conserving surgery, approximately 50 percent of DCIS that recur locally (in the same breast) do so as invasive breast cancer, and in these recurrences the invasive component carries the same risks as other invasive cancers. One might logically argue that if mastectomy gave a 100 percent cure rate then most patients should opt for mastectomy. However, most patients with DCIS can now expect to be cured with a segmental resection, if local radiation treatment is added. Many women and their doctors believe the advantages of breast-conserving surgery outweigh mastectomy even if the chance of cure is slightly less than 100 percent. Even radiation treatment is not always necessary to achieve cure. Many patients can expect complete cure with segmental resection only, if they have low-grade tumors and clear surgical margins. Information gained from clinical trials on large numbers of patients help doctors select the optimal treatment for individual patients. Many patients with DCIS will still need mastectomy, but it is now easier to identify which ones.

A few variables identify which DCISs are likely to recur locally, become invasive, and acquire the potential to metastasize. These bad prognostic variables are[4,5] large size, high nuclear grade, and tumor contamination of the surgical excision margins.

Obviously, the surgeon has no control over the first two of these, but he or she can excise the tumor with a margin of normal breast tissue. Some tumors spread more widely within the breast than even the most meticulous surgeon can predict. If this happens, more surgery can remove additional margins to ensure that they are negative. Sometimes pathologic examination may show more tumor than was apparent during surgery and a subsequent mastectomy will be necessary to ensure negative margins. Postoperative radiotherapy may be successful in eradicating small numbers of tumor cells inadvertently left at the margins.

A woman may reasonably ask, "If the margins are clear, am I guaranteed it will not come back?" Unfortunately, there are no absolute guarantees. Even if the DCIS is completely removed, a new DCIS (or an invasive cancer) may arise from nearby ducts. Whatever caused the first cancer could theoretically cause a second cancer. Nevertheless, for the 36,000 American women who have DCIS diagnosed every year the prognosis is excellent. With a high degree of confidence they can expect to be cured. A recurrence a few years later will bring back all the fears that terrified the woman the first-time cancer was diagnosed. It is thoroughly demoralizing. Nevertheless, even at this stage the patient is eminently curable.

Regarding lobular carcinoma in situ, if it is discovered incidentally in a biopsy specimen removed for benign disease, there is no evidence to suggest that a patient will benefit from further surgery. If it is discovered in association with invasive cancer or DCIS, treatment and prognosis is determined by these other components.[6]

Unlike carcinoma in situ, invasive cancer metastasizes and kills. Prognosticating for individual patients with invasive cancer is often difficult. Knowledge about which tumors are more dangerous gives oncologists an opportunity to treat these more aggressively. To treat all breast cancers with maximum aggressiveness would be unjustifiable; many thousands of patients would receive unnecessary treatment. Such treatment would not help most patients, would seriously harm many, and would kill some.

Medical scientists have probably studied a hundred or more variables that influence prognosis. Many carry either a good or a bad outcome risk. Detailed study often shows that these variables are strongly associated with each other and they all give the same information (i.e., they are co-dependent). Let's use a simple example to illustrate this idea.

Suppose we wanted to know what were the factors influencing an American boy's height. Most of us with a spark of common sense would realize that it was the boy's age. We would also accept that nutrition, possibly ethnic factors, and the parents' height were also important. However, suppose that we decided to study, among other things, various bits of anatomy. We would find that there was a strong correlation between height and the length of the leg, and possibly the diameter of the leg, the length of the forearm, and so on. It is probable that after studying 100 boys we could measure just the upper arm and predict accurately a boys' height—most of the time.

This example shows that all the measurements are so tightly co-dependent that any one of them gives the information we need. It is likely that by studying a boy's height at intervals, say yearly from age one to ten, the trend would predict with reasonable accuracy height at age 16. In the example above, each of the measurements (variables) would help us predict the outcome. These will not be independent variables, as they all give us more or less the same information. One of the measurements, e.g., leg length, might be the strongest predictor and we would say that this was an independent predictor and all the other measurements were not independent. However, other parts of our study might show that nutrition or ethnic origin are also separate independent variables. Now, by measuring three separate independent predictors we should get more accurate information. Even so, our predictions would be wrong sometimes.

Likewise, we try to predict cancer outcome by measuring the most important variables (if we can identify them). Studies that look at one variable at a time and correlate these with the final outcome are easy to perform and are called univariate analyses. Studies that look at the co-dependency of many variables are complicated and are called multivariate analyses. In general, for cancer prognostication, only multivariate analyses are useful. The most powerful independent prognostic indicator for invasive breast cancer (and for most other cancers) is the stage, or extent of spread, at the time of diagnosis. Staging attempts to quantify the extent of tumor bulk and how far it has spread. One common staging system is the TNM system. T stands for tumor characteristics (usually the size), N stands for lymph node metastases, and M stands for distant metastases. Tumor staging protocols get revised regularly, with minor modifications. Depending on a combination of tumor size and the extent of lymph node or distant metastases the tumor is staged as follows:

• Stage 1. Cancers 2 cm or less without nodal involvement and no distant metastases.

• Stage 2. Cancers 5 cm or less with involved but clinically movable axillary nodes and no distant metastases. Cancers greater than 5 cm with no lymph node and no distant metastases are also in Stage 2.

• Stage 3. Cancers greater than 5 cm with lymph node metastases.

• Stage 4. Cancer has metastasized to distant organs (e.g. bone, lungs, liver, brain).

There are also some modifications of these criteria in special circumstances.

Within each stage there are various substages. There are also other staging systems and classifications, but they all more or less give the same information.

The term Stage 0 is used for DCIS without invasion.

If a woman with Stage 1 breast cancer has a mastectomy, in theory the cancer is gone; she should be cured and logically should not need any further treatment. In practice, it is not quite like that. When we say someone has Stage 1 cancer, what we are really saying is that our tests and measurements show no evidence of spread outside the breast. That is not the same as saying it has not spread, only that we could not find any tumor elsewhere. For most patients, when we say a tumor is Stage 1 disease we are correct. The patient will survive. If a few tumor cells break away from the main tumor they can hide in lymph nodes or other tissues and remain undetected. Tumor cells usually spread first to the lymph nodes and later by the bloodstream to other organs. This is not always the case. Sometimes tumor cells get into the bloodstream before going to lymph nodes; with small, well-differentiated, low-grade tumors, this is rare.

Why is pathologic examination of the lymph nodes not 100 percent accurate? There are many reasons. Some lymph nodes are never examined. The axilla contains important structures other than lymph nodes—in particular, blood vessels and nerves supplying the muscles and tissues of the arm. Lymph nodes lie hidden between these structures, camouflaged by mounds of fat. A surgeon doesn't just look into the armpit and neatly pick out lymph nodes. Node removal requires meticulous dissection. Most surgeons do not remove all the lymph nodes—the more he removes the greater the risk of damaging other structures. In most hospitals, the surgeon leaves some nodes behind. These are not examined pathologically. In theory, these could harbor some hidden metastases. However, we know that statistically a sample of five or more lymph nodes gives the same information as a complete dissection, and it is much safer. Some highly skilled surgeons still argue that complete axillary dissection is useful. Most cancer experts do not agree.

The thinking behind axillary dissection has advanced remarkably in the past five years. We know that axillary dissection does not improve patient survival.[78] Its value is the staging information it gives. Not so long ago, we thought that complete or near-complete axillary dissection was necessary for accurate staging. We now know complete dissection is not necessary for staging. Axillary sampling gives the same information. It appears then that the risk of missing pathologically identifiable tumor by leaving behind some lymph nodes is real but small. It is beginning to look as if biopsy of just one or two axillary nodes may give the same information—not just any lymph node, but the sentinel node.[9,10]

As its name suggests, the sentinel is the first node that guards the entry to the rest of the axillary nodes (Figure 8.1). The theory behind using this node is simple. If tumor cells are going into the axilla they will enter the sentinel node first. We assume that if they go there some of them will remain there while others progress to the deeper nodes. Logically, if tumor cells are not in the sentinel node, then the other nodes are also negative.

In theory, examination of the sentinel node gives the required staging information. Clinical trials will tell us if this is also true in practice. Patients are node positive, or node negative. This information allows medical oncologists to decide on the best chemotherapy regimen. At present (year 2001) very few centers have extensive experience with sentinel node biopsy. To identify the sentinel node, the surgeon injects a tracer dye or a radioactive tracer into the tumor, just before surgery. During surgery, the sentinel node takes up the dye or radioactive material. The dye stains the sentinel node and the surgeon can identify it visually. He can identify the lymph node containing the radioactive tracer with a Geiger counter. There are many ongoing international studies looking at how reliable sentinel node biopsy is, and how best this technique might be used. Initial studies suggest it is highly reliable.

The lymph nodes we examine are in the axilla. However, there are other lymph nodes draining the breast. These are within the chest cavity (the thorax) and we do not examine them. Metastases may remain here undetected. In the past, some enthusiastic surgeons used to split the rib cage to dissect these nodes. After some time and study, it became obvious that this painful procedure was a waste of time and gave little additional useful information.

Getting back to the axillary dissection and axillary sampling—even with a complete axillary dissection the pathologist may fail to detect a few tumor cells. Standard surgical pathology practice is to "sample" each lymph node—usually along its greatest diameter. It is not feasible to "completely" examine every axillary lymph node. Each histology section is only four microns in thickness (this is less than the thickness of one cell). Complete examination of the axillary nodes would generate approximately 9,000 glass slides. For some small laboratories that might represent six months' work. We know from the studies of some rather obsessive pathologists that even if we examined every minute piece of tissue in every lymph node, we would not get enough useful information to justify such a mammoth task. The statistics from such studies indicate that sampling each node gives the same information as complete examination.

Even if we could reliably identify every tumor cell in every lymph node, we still would get the staging wrong occasionally. Sometimes tumor cells get directly into the bloodstream and bypass the lymph nodes. Some patients with negative nodes will have distant metastases at the time of diagnosis. These can be detected if they are large. It they are microscopic they cannot. In practice, unless the patient has symptoms referable to distant organs most clinicians will not order sophisticated staging procedures (and healthy insurance organizations will not pay for these). Surgeons sometimes order a small number of "metastatic tests" for patients with high-risk (large, high-grade) tumors. These tests are usually chest x-ray, bone scan, ultrasound examination of the liver, and biochemical tests of liver function.

At the time of diagnosis, for the purposes of treatment and prognostication, most patients fall into two main groups—node positive and node negative. The node positive group can be further categorized on the basis of the extent of positivity. Statistically, those patients with four or fewer involved nodes do better than those with more than four involved. Other factors may also be important, such as whether the nodes contain only tiny microscopic foci (micrometastases) or more bulky metastases. Some experts also argue that if the nodal metastases extend beyond the lymph node capsule into surrounding tissue, this also adversely affects prognosis. The evidence for this is not convincing.

The niceties of quantitative nodal involvement are rapidly becoming less important as oncologists devise better chemotherapy regimens. Not so long ago, they did not treat node-negative patients with chemotherapy. Newer studies show that some Stage 1 patients benefit from newer chemotherapeutic regimens.[7]

Regardless of the methodology we use, we fail to detect some micrometastases. Therefore we can ask, "Are there any clues in the primary tumor that help predict prognosis?" The answer is yes, there are many. These are somewhat analogous to many of the measurements used in the example above to predict the boy's height. Most are related to each other, and pathologists, biochemists, and molecular biologists have studied these prognostic variables extensively. As each new test becomes available they compare it with existing data to see if it adds any new useful information. In other words, scientists and biostatisticians check to see if it is an independent prognostic variable.

It is common practice to find that many prognostic tests appear very promising initially, but subsequently fall into disuse. Studies in reputable international journals often raise expectations that some new enzyme, hormone receptor, or genetic change will be of great benefit in stratifying patients into particular risk groups. When the studies are repeated in multiple laboratories, under differing conditions, and in different groups of patients, their initial promise falters. Regrettably, most of these tests end up gathering dust.

The one variable, other than stage, that has withstood the test of time more than any other is tumor grade. This is by no means perfect and has many detractors and critics. As explained in chapter four, a grade is assigned using three microscopic features—the extent of gland formation (differentiation), the degree of nuclear abnormality (pleomorphism—a measure of the amount of abnormal DNA in the cell) and the number of mitoses present (a measure of tumor growth rate) (Figure 4.5). Like the newer tests mentioned above, grade too suffers from lack of reproducibility. However, it is more reproducible and more useful than most other tests. Pathologists who have participated in training programs specifically for grading show a high level of accuracy and interobserver agreement. Grading requires no sophisticated equipment, just a microscope and a well-trained pathologist, and a little patience. It is quick, relatively simple and inexpensive. More importantly, it is useful. Tumors are graded 1, 2 or 3, corresponding to low, intermediate, or high-grade. Grade one tumors have the best prognosis and grade 3 the worst. Most existing treatment and prognostic protocols use grade as an important piece of data. For example node-negative patients with small low grade invasive tumors usually do not require or benefit from chemotherapy, whereas those node-negative patients with high grade tumors may benefit.[7] This rationale is based on the knowledge that grade 3 tumors often metastasize whereas grade 1 tumors do so infrequently.

Using other techniques such as immunohistochemistry, radiolabeled antibody tagging, flow cytometry or PCR (polymerase chain reaction, see page 117) researchers can detect tumor cells in lymph nodes. Such procedures may prove useful in the future for more definitive staging strategies. At present, standard lymph node staging in most reputable institutions throughout the world consists of axillary node sampling (four or more lymph nodes) followed by routine pathologic (microscopic) examination. Still, we know that this standard will miss some metastases, although rarely.

Might New Research Techniques Give Us Better Prognostic Information?

The harder you look, the more you will find. Using new molecular biology techniques, in particular the polymerase chain reaction (PCR), medical scientists can find a single metastatic tumor cell in lymph nodes that appear free of tumor by other methods. Like a powerful magnet looking for a needle in a haystack, PCR can fish out one tumor cell hiding among 100,000 normal cells. PCR can also find single cells in the bone marrow, identifying distant metastases when none would be expected. Such awesome technology also poses serious problems. We base our therapeutic strategies on well founded, proven results from clinical trials. There are no clear guidelines yet about what should be done in a situation where standard tests are negative for metastases and PCR shows micrometastases. A recent study in the New England Journal of Medicine confirms that so-called minimal residual disease adversely affects the prognosis for patients with colon cancer.[11] It is likely that new studies will show the same for breast cancer.[12-14] As their value becomes widely accepted and appreciated, some of what we now classify as research techniques will become part of routine oncology practice in the 21st century. Clinical trials will evaluate and probably confirm their usefulness.

Because tumor grading relies on experience, training, and to some extent the pathologist's patience, many consider it too subjective. Why not get computers to analyze tumor cells and identify more consistently what the human eye can do? By training a computer to analyze histology sections through a camera attached to a microscope it could measure differentiation, nuclear size, nuclear pleomorphism, and many additional features the human brain could not possibly recognize. This approach, known as quantitative computerized image analysis, is theoretically excellent. In some areas of pathology it is already proving very useful. This technology is now available and in use for cervical cytology screening.[15,16] Numerous small research studies show that image analysis is also useful in breast cancer. Computers can measure what percentage of cells within a tumor is dividing and how many are resting. They can also measure the total DNA and chromosomal content in tumor cells. However, there are also many conflicting studies showing that this approach is not yet acceptable as a clinical tool. A pathologist's eye-brain combination is still better than the camera-computer combination.

Flow cytometry uses a different type of computer technology. It too measures DNA and chromosomal content and quantifies the degree of tumor cell abnormality. It can also measure the s–phase of the dividing cells. Flow cytometry gives important information concerning how rapidly tumor cells are growing. In turn, this gives prognostic information. However, like computerized image analysis, and despite early promise, flow cytometry is rarely used in routine breast pathology practice. It is however, very useful in the assessment of patients with leukemia and lymphoma.

In the future, some of these computer methods may replace microscopy, or certain aspects of microscopy. This is not likely to happen soon. Many factors contribute to the computer's difficulties. First, there is tumor heterogeneity. If you examine a tumor microscopically, you will often find that all parts of the tumor do not look the same. As you move from microscopic field to microscopic field you will find that in some areas glands are well formed, whereas in other areas they are poorly formed or nonexistent. In other words, some areas are well- and others are poorly differentiated, or undifferentiated. A pathologist can examine ten or more histology slides representing an entire cross-sectional area of the tumor. He or she can do this in a few minutes and then decide which area is most suitable for grading (the least differentiated area). It would take a computer hours to do the same task. It is technically difficult to feed a flow cytometer or a computer with the correct tumor cells from the most appropriate part of the tumor. In other words, the results would be unreliable due to sampling errors. The computer data from different areas of a tumor would reflect the underlying structure but would be almost impossible to interpret intelligently. As technology improves, this may all change.

The second major problem the computer has is the inability of its software to discriminate between touching and overlapping cells. Computers still have a long way to go to match the capability of the trained eyes and brain when it comes to identifying cells in histology sections. Imagine you are looking at a garden full of flowers—all more or less the same color, and more or less the same shape. Let's say they are all red roses. A toddler with normal three-dimensional vision would have no difficulty identifying individual flowers. Now, take a photograph of this garden, or a part of it, for example a small cluster of roses. Even the most sophisticated computer will have great difficulty separating and identifying each flower in a two-dimensional picture. Computers can learn to do this. However, to do so accurately, they need constant coaxing from an expert programmer sitting at their keyboards. In contrast, the human eye and brain can readily interpret the three-dimensional spatial relationship between the flowers. The idea in getting computers to give reproducible reliable data is to get them to do it without human interference. Apart from cervical cytology, they still have a long way to go. Nevertheless, as hardware gets faster and software improves, computers may give the same information that an expert pathologist gets from the microscope. This will not happen soon.

One group of markers has found a routine use in clinical practice—hormone receptors. While pathologists are still arguing about the best method for measuring them, all cancer experts agree that their presence or absence gives useful therapeutic and prognostic information.[7,17-19] The hormones estrogen and progesterone influence the growth of normal breast epithelial cells. Hormones bind to the cell surface by clinging to specific receptors. Analogous to a lock and key mechanism, the hormone is the key and the receptor is the lock. Once bound to the cell surface, estrogen and progesterone can enter the cell and turn on various cell growth switches. Many breast cancers have hormone receptors, and estrogen stimulates these tumor cells to grow. Better differentiated tumors tend to have the most receptors and undifferentiated tumors tend to have few or none. This turns out to be a useful piece of information with therapeutic implications. For decades surgeons knew that ovarian hormones influenced breast cancer growth. In order to control growth, they sometimes removed the ovaries (oophorectomy) to get rid of estrogen. They also radiated the pituitary gland that stimulated the ovaries to secrete estrogen. (The pituitary gland sits at the base of the brain.) If you could block estrogen from binding to cell receptors you would achieve the same effect as oophorectomy. There is a drug that does this called Tamoxifen. Oncologists use Tamoxifen for patients whose tumor cells are covered by estrogen-binding receptors. For the past 20 years, biochemists measured estrogen receptors, using complicated sophisticated techniques. Now, almost every pathology department can measure estrogen receptors directly in histology sections, using relatively easy immunohistochemistry techniques. However, not every pathology department does this, usually because of lack of financial resources.

Another group of markers tries to identify damaged genes. Altered genes control every aspect of tumor growth—its structure, its ability to destroy normal tissue, and its ability to metastasize. Normal genes send signals that instruct cells to behave themselves. Damaged genes lose normal control mechanisms. If we could identify which genes are causing what, we should be able to predict which tumors will behave badly. As molecular biology developed, scientists identified more and more cell-controlling genes. They began to study these genes in all cancers, including breast cancer. They found hundreds of abnormalities. But, just as there is heterogeneity in the microscopic appearance, there is also genetic heterogeneity within tumors. Different pieces of the same tumor have different genetic abnormalities, and often these vary from tumor to tumor. We have now identified so many genetic changes in breast cancer that it is difficult to know which are the important ones.

Which genetic mutations contribute to cancer growth and which are the innocent bystanders? Which ones drive cells wild and out of control? Despite the widespread genetic chaos lurking within tumor DNA, it is gradually becoming clear that some mutations contribute more than others to growth, invasion, and metastasis.[20] Identifying these may help us prognosticate. At present, the main contenders are the p53, nm23, mdm2, HER-2/neu, and a handful of others.[21-23] Earlier researchers looked for a single gene defect to explain all of a tumor's behavior. We no longer believe that a lone villain is to blame. It is far more likely that a Mafia of genetic defects acts in unison to control tumor behavior. It is not yet clear if there is a unique leader among them. If there is, p53 is the likely godfather.

As mentioned earlier, tumor growth depends on factors other than cell division or proliferation. Most normal cells die at a constant rate. This is apoptosis. Tumor cells often do not die at a normal rate. They accumulate and contribute to the tumor bulk. In many tumors damaged genes lose control of normal apoptosis. Abnormalities in these proliferative and apoptotic genes correlate with prognosis. However, like so many other tests, they give inconsistent and conflicting results. This inconsistency means that they are not suitable for routine monitoring or prognostication. Nevertheless, one of these has proven more helpful than others, namely HER-2/neu.[24] This gene codes for a growth-promoting protein embedded in the outer layer of each tumor cell. Its presence correlates with aggressive behavior and it is present in many high grade tumors. A new drug treatment uses antibodies directed against these proteins and stops tumor cell growth. Early trials with this drug (Herceptin) are promising.[25-27] In March 1998, the FDA approved Herceptin for clinical use in patients with advanced cancer. It is too early to say how useful it will be for other patients. Also, its safety in patients with less advanced disease is still unknown.

During the past decade new insights into tumor angiogenesis gave us ample opportunity to study the relationship between angiogenesis and prognosis. Many studies demonstrated such a correlation.[28,29] For technical reasons, quantification of angiogenesis as a prognostic "test" or marker is not in widespread use. This "test" has been around for over ten years and occupies numerous pages of mainstream medical journals. Nevertheless, the fact that most cancer workers do not measure angiogenesis probably means that they find it unhelpful or just too difficult and complicated to use.

Some tumors vanish rapidly with chemotherapy. Some do not. Why? There are many possible reasons. One fascinating finding from molecular biology and pharmacology studies is that these tumors can prevent drugs from entering their cells. Furthermore, if the drugs do manage to get inside the cell they are quickly ejected. These cells are resistant to chemotherapy. Scientists now understand how they do this. These tumor cells have activated a group of genes known as multidrug-resistant (MDR) genes.[30,31] These genes produce a protein that guards the cell wall and rapidly evicts drugs as they try to gain entry. Tumors that express a high level of MDR genes are resistant to therapy and have a poorer prognosis than those not expressing the gene.

Although research techniques offer great promise for the future, in everyday practice, surgeons and oncologists try to prognosticate as best they can, using tumor stage and histologic grade. As mentioned above, while far from perfect, they are the best we have for routine, consistent, and practical use.

In summary, the most important factors affecting prognosis are:

DCIS
— There is almost 100 percent chance of cure.

Chance of local recurrence depends on:
- Status of surgical margins
- Postoperative radiation therapy
- Tumor grade

LCIS found incidentally:
— No special treatment required.

DCIS or **LCIS** found in association with invasive cancer
— Prognosis depends on the invasive cancer.

INVASIVE CANCER
— Local recurrence is the same as for DCIS above.
  Long-term survival depends on:
  - Stage at time of diagnosis
  - Tumor size
  - Tumor grade
  - Whether or not the tumor is estrogen receptor positive

Tumor type is also important for some patients. For example, tubular carcinomas have an excellent (greater that 90 percent 5-year survival prognosis). Tubular carcinoma is a special type of well differentiated, low-grade (grade 1) carcinoma.

As mentioned above, there are many other variables that affect prognosis. However, these are considered mostly in a research setting and do not play a major role in day-to-day clinical practice.

Information Highway: Where to Find Everything You Need to Know

Knowledge is of two kinds. We know a subject ourselves, or we know where we can find information on it.
— *Samuel Johnson*

What do patients with breast cancer want to know? They want to know what treatment they will get, how it will affect them, and if it will cure them. Some patients want to know the details; most want an overview and an explanation of the most important points. A few leave everything in the hands of the surgeon and a higher power.

How much information they need depends on many factors, but mostly it depends on their education, their attitude toward life, and their previous experience with friends and family, and possibly their age. Many patients will know relatives or friends who have had breast, colon, or other cancers. Some of these may have made astonishing recoveries; some will have died. Some will have gone through intensive chemotherapy unscathed; some will have suffered months of fatigue and nausea. Some will have had pain.

Avid readers will remember stories in women's magazines about the courage and resilience of movie stars, singers, or politicians. They will remember documentaries and news clips that hyped scientific "breakthroughs," gene therapy, and new wonder drugs. The media bombard us with cancer stories, and many of them are about breast cancer. Messages are often conflicting and leave lay people, who do not know how to separate medical reality from scientific fancy, confused.

Patients may have difficulty understanding medical principles but they will not have any difficulty understanding the crucial differences between breast-conserving surgery and mastectomy, between radiotherapy and no radiotherapy, or between chemotherapy and no chemotherapy.

The immediate source of information is the patient's doctor and medical team. Every year, surgeons, nurses, radiotherapists, and oncologists treat hundreds of breast cancer patients. They know the problems patients face. They know the experiences of previous patients. They know what helped them and what did not. At least, they know and understand medical problems. However, many doctors may not have great interest or insight into some of the patients' non-medical anxieties—about their sexuality, about conflicts at home, or about problems with neighbors and friends.

Social workers attached to cancer units can help greatly. Many patients want to talk to other patients about their experiences. Patient support groups, often sponsored by local cancer societies, provide encouragement and information. Governments or government-funded agencies provide extensive cancer information. The National Cancer Institute and many other organizations provide clear, written information on dozens of cancers, including breast cancer. Unfortunately, most patients do not know this information exists. Even if they know the information is out there, they do not know how to find it.

Angela Coulter, director of policy and development at the King's Fund in London, writing in the British Medical Journal, describes how shared decision-making helps patients. She says, "Patients with breast cancer suffer less depression and anxiety if they are treated by doctors who adopt a participative consultation style." Patients can participate better in decision making if they are well informed.

Bookstores and libraries have medical sections, and usually some cancer books. Because breast cancer is so common they invariably carry books on the topic. These are mostly self-help books and sometimes they are useful. Unfortunately they are often out of date. Sometimes they give unrealistic hope when they explain that diets and exercise can cure patients. Medical libraries carry excellent books on every aspect of breast cancer. These books are useful for doctors and medical students but they are useless for the layperson, as they are far too technical. Also, only major cities have medical schools and their libraries are not readily accessible to local citizens.

Without doubt, the outstanding source of cancer information is the Internet. The pages of the World Wide Web are filled with more useful (and useless) information than most medical school libraries. This information covers everything from pure basic science to detailed descriptions of different chemotherapy protocols, their side effects, benefits, and complications. It lists e-mail addresses and contact phone numbers for cancer support groups throughout the world. Patients talk to each other on chat lines. Doctors answer questions. It advises doctors also and presents them with timely updates on all aspects of cancer care. It informs doctors in doctor-talk and gives patients the same information in nontechnical patient-talk. It shows before and after treatment photographs, x-rays, mammograms, CT and MRI scans, and pathology specimens. The World Wide Web has information on every medical condition imaginable, from the rarest genetic disorder to the most trivial skin rash. Its cancer coverage is particularly good and some web sites are outstanding. Many have won media awards not just for their content, but also for their presentation.

In mid–1999, the Internet listed 15,000 medical web sites, and they are growing monthly. Most have sections on cancer and almost all of these have a section on breast cancer. It is difficult to know which ones provide the most useful information for an individual patient. However a few deserve special mention. My own favorites are Oncolink and Intelihealth. The University of Pennsylvania Cancer Center sponsors Oncolink, and Aetna U.S. Healthcare and Johns Hopkins University and Health System sponsors Intelihealth. Their addresses:

http://oncolink.upenn.edu/
http://www.intelihealth.com/IH/ihtIH

Some web sites are breast disease or breast cancer sites only. These are updated regularly, often weekly or even daily. The wonderful thing about this web information is that for the most part, it is accurate, comprehensive, presented in a way that anyone can understand, and it is free.

Those interested in tracking new information can subscribe to medical information news updates provided by news agencies such as Reuters or the major television networks. Some of these charge for their services, many do not. Some sites claim that medical school doctors check their information before they put it on the web. Some sites (e.g., InteliHealth) will email you automatically with an update on your topic of choice, whenever they get new information. And they do it for free. The Reuters address: http://www.reutershealth.com/.

Doctors and the public have free access to an amazing database called Medline. The National Library of Medicine can claim the credit for this unique source of information. This database contains information on every major medical article published since the early 1960s. If the article appeared in any important medical or scientific journal, in any part of the world, it is referenced here. Furthermore, most references contain a summary of the article in English, regardless of the language in which it was originally written. The address: http://www.ncbi.nlm.nih.gov/PubMed/.

Although Medline contains the most complete medical database available anywhere, its contents and messages are difficult to decipher unless you are a medic or a scientist. It is not written in the layman's language. In fact, for the non-medical reader it would be difficult to find the most relevant information for a particular patient. Taken out of context, the information in this database could do more psychological harm than good.

Cancer organizations and doctors often warn patients that there is a lot of wrong and harmful information scattered throughout the Internet. These include references to fraudulent miracle cures. A desperate patient will try anything. In the past, the traveling medicine man with his colored, flavored water sold his cure and moved on. He could not be tracked down. Now, similar medicine men peddle their useless medicines on the Internet and take money from cancer patients and their relatives.

In general, it is a good idea to get your cancer information fromcancer organizations, universities, and medical centers. The following web site will help readers find fraudulent medical claims: http://www.quackwatch.com/.

The Internet provides many ways for finding the information you need. If you have not used computers before you will need a few hours' instruction on the basics. Consider taking night classes in your area or asking a friend or relative (or one of the local kids) to get you started. If you have used a computer before but have not used the Internet, it should take about 30 minutes to get the hang of things. The Internet provider will charge you for use on a weekly, monthly or yearly basis or with some other time-related formula. More recently, some Internet providers are offering free access, claiming they can make their money from advertising. Once you have access to the Internet most of the information is free. In many countries, users will have to pay local telephone call rates while they are online.

The end of this chapter contains the World Wide Web addresses to a number of breast cancer sites. There are many others. Finding them is as simple as typing "breast cancer" into one of the "search engines."

A search engine is a piece of software that searches for web sites depending on the words or phrases you type onto the screen. It is like looking in a dictionary, except that instead of searching for the explanation of words it searches for the addresses you need. When the addresses appear on the screen you click on whichever one you require and the magic of the Internet whisks you to its site. From here you follow whatever links stimulate your interest.

To start this searching process you begin with the search engine. There are many search engines. The best known are Yahoo!, WebCrawler, Excite, Google, and HotBot. Their addresses are at the end of this chapter.

When you first log on to the Internet, chances are you will probably be using one of the two main "browsers," Internet Explorer or Netscape. Browsers are free programs that let you move about the World Wide Web—they allow you to browse the information. These browsers have icons (small pictures) or buttons in the top section of the screen that automatically start one of the search engines when you click on it.

Below is an example of the beginning of a search on breast cancer (Figure 10.1). In the first view, I typed "breast cancer" into the search space in the WebCrawler search engine. Within a few seconds this returned a selection of possible addresses (Figure 10.2). I chose Oncolink and the next figure shows the beginning of the result from Oncolink (Figure 10.3). Some websites show visitors where they can find commercial services to find the information, for a fee.

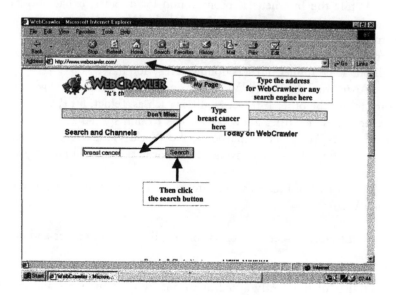

Figure 10.1. WebCrawler 1

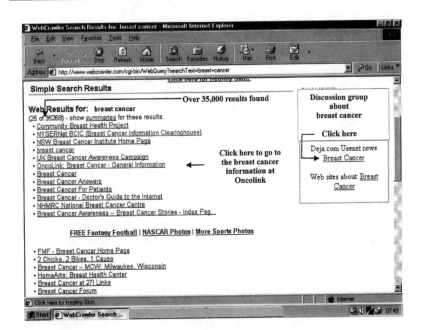

Figure 10.2. WebCrawler 2

While the Internet has been around for decades, it has only been available to the general public since World Wide Web browsers were introduced in the mid–90s. In 1990 there were 300,000 Internet users, worldwide. In 1994 this figure grew to 4 million, and in 1998 it was 65 million. The number of users doubles every 100 days.

Apart from the World Wide Web and email, most patients will rarely want to use the other Internet facilities such as Telnet, FTP, Gopher, or Archie. These facilities allow researchers to find specialized documents or programs. For practical purposes, the World Wide Web gives access to more information than anyone, doctor or patient, could possibly want or need.

What sort of breast cancer information can you find on the World Wide Web?

• the latest research information on all aspects of cancer and breast cancer

• explanations of surgical operations and procedures

• lists of frequently asked questions by other patients and expert answers

• politics and events relating to breast cancer

- direct chat with other patients
- new treatments, e.g., bone marrow and stem cell transplants
- side effects and complications of treatments
- social impact—home, sexuality, finance, costs
- tips on how to cope with general and specific problems
- psychological support
- updates on clinical trials
- news items as they break

If you wish to read what other people have written about breast cancer books, you can do so at the Amazon book store on the web (http://www.amazon.com). This site gives a summary of most books and how their readers rated them. It is a fascinating web site.

If you do not have the time or interest to learn how to use computers or the Internet, then professional information finders will get information for you, for a fee. These are commissioned searches and their uses have pros and cons. In general it is no longer necessary to use such agencies as the information on the Internet is so good and so easy to find. For information on the advantages and disadvantages of using a medical search service, see http://www.cancerguid.org/search_service.html.

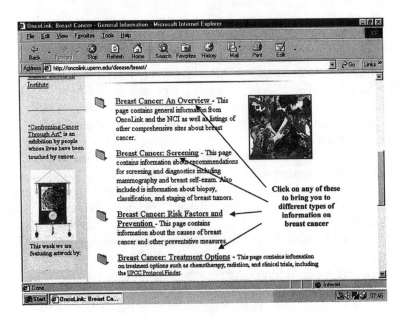

Figure 10.3. WebCrawler 3

Search engines

Ask Jeeves, http://www.askjeeves.com/index.asp
Google, http://www.google.com/
Yahoo!, http://www.yahoo.com/
Excite, http://www.excite.com/
HotBot, http://hotbot.lycos.com/
Infoseek, http://www.go.com/
AltaVista, http://www.altavista.com/
WebCrawler, http://www.webcrawler.com/

Web sites

American Cancer Society, http://www.cancer.org/
Association of Cancer Online Resources, http://www.acor.org/
Cancer news, http://www.cancernews.com/breast.htm
Cancer statistics, National Cancer Institute home page, http://www.nci.nih.gov/
Oncolink breast cancer page from the University of Pennsylvania Cancer Center,   http://oncolink.upenn.edu/disease/breast/
List of addresses to other breast cancer sites with hypertext links, http://www.webmed.com/spotlight/brcancer.html
InteliHealth home page, http://www.intelihealth.com/

Books

Nancy G. Brinker and Catherine McEvilly Harris. The Race Is Run One Step at a Time: Every Woman's Guide to Taking Charge of Breast Cancer and My Personal Story. Summit Publication Group, 1995.

Rob Buckman. What You Really Need to Know About Cancer. London: Macmillan, 1996.

Peter A. Dervan. Understanding Cancer: A Scientific and Clinical Guide for the Layperson. McFarland & Company, 1999.

Susan Diemert Moch and Allan Graubard. Breast Cancer: Twenty Women's Stories: Becoming More Alive Through the Experience. Jones & Bartlett, 1999.

Yashar Hirshaut, Peter I. Pressman, and Amy S. Langer. Breast Cancer: The Complete Guide. Bantam Books, 1997.

Ronnie Kaye. Spinning Straw into Gold: Your Emotional Recovery from Breast Cancer. Fireside, 1991.

Judy C. Kneece. Helping Your Mate Face Breast Cancer: Tips for Becoming an Effective Support Partner for the One You Love During the Breast Cancer Experience. Edu Care Inc., 1995.

Vladimir Lange. Be a Survivor: Your Guide to Breast Cancer Treatment. Lange Productions, 1998.

Kathy Latour. The Breast Cancer Companion. Avon Books, 1994.

John Link. Breast Cancer Survival Manual: A Step-by-Step Guide for the Woman with Newly Diagnosed Breast Cancer. Owl Books, 1998.

Susan Love and Karen Lindsey. Dr. Susan Love's Breast Book. 3rd edition. Addison Wesley, 2000.

Margit Esser Porter (editor), et al. Hope Is Contagious: The Breast Cancer Treatment Survival Handbook. Fireside, 1997.

Lillie Shockney. Breast Cancer Survivors' Club: A Nurse's Experience. Windsor House, 1997.

Bruce Sokol. Breast Cancer : A Husband's Story. Crane Hill, 1997.

Marisa C. Weiss and Ellen Weiss. Living Beyond Breast Cancer: A Survivor's Guide for When Treatment Ends and the Rest of Your Life Begins. Times Books, 1998.

Rebecca Zuckweiler. Living in the Postmastectomy Body: Learning to Live in and Love Your Body Again. Andrews McMeel Publishing, 1998.

The Future

As the 21st century begins, doctors are winning the war against AIDS. Unfortunately, it is not easy to see a similar victory against breast cancer. However, we can take heart from the AIDS story. A few years ago, scientists and doctors where pessimistic. Suddenly, a breakthrough in treatment changed the future for AIDS patients and new treatments have removed the death sentence that threatened all AIDS patients. The future for these patients is far brighter in the 21st century. Nevertheless, experts warn us against the dangers of complacency. The war against AIDS is not over yet.[1] Cancer specialists hope for a similar breakthrough for their patients. However, theirs is a more difficult war. With AIDS, we know the cause: HIV (the human immunodeficiency virus). Unlike AIDS, with breast cancer we do not know the enemy, or if there are many enemies, and until we know this, the best we can do is to try and identify risk factors and eliminate them.

Although we cannot prevent breast cancer, we can reduce the toll it takes on individuals and society. We can do this by improving our understanding of how it grows and spreads, by diagnosing it at an early curable stage, and by improving treatment.

The epidemiology detectives continue their search for links between breast cancer and environmental hazards. Meanwhile, laboratory scientists check tumor cells to see what drives them, and how they differ from normal cells. The scientifically developed nations spend billions of dollars trying to identify the mechanisms that control cancer cells. Scientists pass this information to their pharmacology colleagues who design new drugs to eliminate or block these mechanisms. This painstaking process of checking and testing goes on daily in laboratories around the globe. Most new drugs never make it to the patient. They prove to be either ineffective or, in preliminary tests, have too many toxic side effects.

Is it possible to prevent cancer in women with a higher than normal risk? Apparently yes—by preventive surgery.[2] This means having both breasts removed. Some patients may choose this option, if they come from a family with a strong history of breast cancer. This is particularly true if they have known mutated genes and there is a history of breast cancer in first-degree relatives (mothers or sisters). As many of these patients are also at risk for ovarian cancer, they may chose to have their ovaries removed, as well as their breasts. However, even prophylactic surgery is not foolproof.[3] Theoretically, tiny fragments of breast tissue may be left behind after surgery and cancers could arise from these.

Less dramatic treatment may prevent cancer in women with smaller risks. Women who already have had one breast cancer are at risk for developing another. Women who have fibrocystic disease with increased proliferation and cellular atypia are also at risk (atypical ductal hyperplasia). There is good evidence the drug Tamoxifen, by blocking the action of estrogen, may prevent cancer in these women.[4-7] Several similar drugs are also undergoing trials.

Some experts encourage women to adopt a healthy lifestyle. Exercise, good diet, weight control, fewer cigarettes, and less alcoholic intake are all associated with a lower incidence of breast cancer. The adoption of a "healthy" lifestyle may prevent cancer in some women, but it is impossible to predict which ones.

The ideal goal is prevention. If that is not possible, early diagnosis is the next best alternative. The best choice for early detection is mammography. However, there is plenty of room for improvement here. Mammography, like all tests, has false positives and false negatives. Radiologists, physicists, and computer scientists are researching new ways to improve diagnosis.[8] These include better ultrasound, computerized interpretation of mammograms, and specialized MRI procedures. The hope is that these will improve diagnosis by improving sensitivity and specificity. In other words, they would find more cancers and reduce the number of women having needless biopsies.

Many tumors secrete tiny quantities of various chemicals. Some cancers, such as cancer of the testis, secrete hormones and chemicals. Biochemists can detect these in blood and urine samples. They are looking for similar markers to help diagnose and monitor breast cancer patients. Such markers would be helpful in identifying whether tumor cells remained in the body after surgery or chemotherapy.[9]

When a heart attack damages heart muscle, an EKG (electrocardiogram) picks up differences in the electrical charge between damaged tissue and surrounding normal tissue. Using similar technology, the EEG (electroencephalogram) detects differences in electrical activity between normal and abnormal brain tissue. Recently, electrophysiologists, using similar technology, have detected several differences between tumor cells and normal breast tissue.[10] The procedure used to identify such changes is harmless and painless. This technology is not sensitive enough to pick up tiny or early cancers, and for the near future will not replace mammography.

The final diagnosis of malignancy still rests with the biopsy, and will continue to do so for many years. At some stage, some molecular biology technique may replace microscopy. However, the pathologist's role as the final decision-maker for cancer diagnosis and grading is assured for the time being. The pathologist's decision-making skills are subjective and depend on knowledge, experience, and pattern recognition. Soon, more objective techniques, such as automated computerized image analysis and image cytometry may complement routine microscopy. These techniques quantify tumor cell size, differentiation, proliferation rates, and measurement of estrogen receptors, cellular oncogenes, and DNA abnormalities. Pathologists already use these computer techniques, but in a research setting. In future, they may use them to help with routine diagnoses.

Better biopsy instruments also contribute to better diagnosis and management. Twenty-five years ago, most surgeons removed tissue for diagnosis with a scalpel, by open biopsy. This required a general anesthetic. Now, they and radiologists mostly use various types of aspiration or cutting needles, and local or no anesthetic is required. Manufacturers and doctors continue to design better instruments for improving the yield of tissue samples and at the same time minimizing patient discomfort.[11]

We can expect improvements in treatment also. Surgeons, radiotherapists, medical oncologists, and their patients participate in clinical trials involving new procedures and new drugs. Every year, thousands of trials test the efficacy of new treatments. Already, some oncologists treat certain patients with stem cell transplants. A few years ago, stem cell transplantation was a radical experimental procedure. Soon, it proved invaluable in the treatment of patients with malignant lymphoma, leukemia, and some other rare diseases. Then oncologists checked its value for selected groups of breast cancer patients. Medical scientists and oncologists argued about the significance of their findings. Some argued that the procedure did not contribute significantly to patient management, and at present the majority opinion is that stem cell transplantation is of unproven value for breast cancer patients. However, for certain groups of cancer patients many oncologists are convinced of its value. Current evidence suggests that stem cell transplantation is not more useful than conventional high dose chemotherapy.[12,13]

Immunologists can teach the body's immune system to recognize certain molecules within its tumors as foreign. In theory, this form of therapy is logical and attractive, but so far results are disappointing. Nevertheless, there are many scientists who believe that immunotherapy when it has advanced a little (or a lot) more will have a definite place alongside, or instead of, conventional chemotherapy.

Vaccines work by stimulating the immune system to recognize and destroy foreign invaders, namely, bacteria and viruses. The purpose of vaccination is to prevent infection. The purpose of cancer immunotherapy is to treat established tumors. Researchers working in the field of immunotherapy hope to teach the immune system to destroy cancer cells.[14–16] Immunotherapy is not new. In the 1890s, William Coley treated cancer patients with bacterial extracts (Coley's toxins). Today's immunotherapists treat patients with tumor extracts. The idea is to modify the tumor cells in some way, such that the patient's immune system recognizes tumor molecules as foreign proteins. If immune cells can do this, there is a good chance that they can destroy the tumor.

To date, immunotherapy has had little success in clinical practice. Those little successes have been mostly with the skin cancer malignant melanoma, and more recently with malignant lymphoma. However, a new immunotherapy drug, Herceptin, is proving beneficial to some breast cancer patients.

Using an antibody that protects against the vicious HER-2/neu oncogene, researchers have recently had some success in breast cancer. This gene makes tumor cells grow rapidly. With the antibody Herceptin, oncologists can block the oncogene, and reduce or prevent tumor growth. After a number of successful clinical trials, the FDA approved Herceptin for patients whose tumors express high levels of HER-2/neu. Oncologists believe this drug is a major breakthrough for some patients.[17,18] Following successful clinical trials, this drug is now available for selected patients.

In a few circumstances, viruses appear to cause cancer. The best examples are hepatitis B virus, which plays a major role in the causation of malignant hepatoma (liver cancer) in certain parts of the word, and human papilloma virus, which appears causally related to cervical cancer. Vaccination against these viruses should prevent hepatoma and cervical cancer.[19–22] This appears to be the case with hepatoma. Vaccination against hepatitis B virus has dramatically reduced the incidence of hepatoma in areas where hepatitis B is endemic. Unfortunately, there is no such vaccine against breast cancer.

For the past decade, immunotherapy has been one of the most intensely investigated areas in cancer therapy. Undoubtedly this will continue. Newer slants on immunotherapy include the use of specific fragments of genes that code for specific antigens; these are DNA vaccines. Presently, most DNA vaccine research is directed toward infectious diseases. However, it is likely that researchers will also investigate their value for cancer patients.[14,23,24]

A greater understanding of tumor cell biology stimulates new treatment ideas. The realization that tumors have their own new blood supply (neoangiogenesis) gave rise to one great idea. If some technique could be found to destroy these blood vessels, tumor cells would be starved of oxygen and nutrients. This stimulated investigators to see if the endothelial cells, lining tumor vessels, had different properties from those lining normal blood vessels. They do.

In turn, this led scientists to search for molecules on the endothelial cells that would bind specifically to toxic drugs. These drugs should destroy the new vessels, and shut down the tumor's nutrient supply lines. At the same time they would leave normal vessels unharmed.

And so, each little discovery led to a new idea. These ideas are now being tested in clinical trials, and scientists (and the media) have become excited about the possibility of anti-angiogenesis therapy. So much so, that one world famous scientist (rashly) said he thought they would have a cure for cancer within two years. The media loved it. His colleagues were quick to dampen enthusiasm by pointing out that this just was not possible within such a timeframe. They were right. Nevertheless, angiogenesis is a logical and attractive target for new forms of treatment.

Gene therapy is a new form of treatment that has captured the public imagination. So far it hasn't cured one cancer patient, and yet the media and funding agencies love it. This treatment has an appealing theoretical basis, and has had a few experimental successes (Figure 11.1). To say

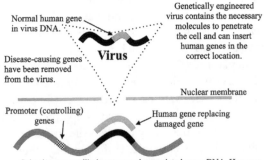

Scientists can readily insert normal genes into human DNA. However, they have not yet succeeded in getting these genes to function normally. Other (promoter) genes control and modify how the main gene works.

Figure 11.1. Gene Therapy

that effective gene therapy for breast cancer patients is light years away is an exaggeration (but only just). There are numerous novel treatments being tested or about to be in the near future (Figures 11.2 and 11.3).

Many critics are quick to point out that scientists are slow in translating new biological information into new treatments. For almost 30 years, various funding agencies have invested billions of dollars in cancer research. The payoff for patients such as those with Hodgkin's disease, testicular cancer, leukemia, and childhood cancers has been dramatic. Most patients with these cancers are now curable. However, for the common adult cancers—lung, breast, prostate, ovary, and colon (as well as

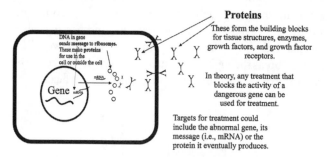

Proteins

These form the building blocks for tissue structures, enzymes, growth factors, and growth factor receptors.

DNA in gene sends message to ribosomes. These make proteins for use in the cell or outside the cell

Gene

In theory, any treatment that blocks the activity of a dangerous gene can be used for treatment.

Targets for treatment could include the abnormal gene, its message (i.e., mRNA) or the protein it eventually produces.

Another possibility is to block the receptors on cells that bind to proteins (Tamoxifen works like this).

mRNA = messenger RNA

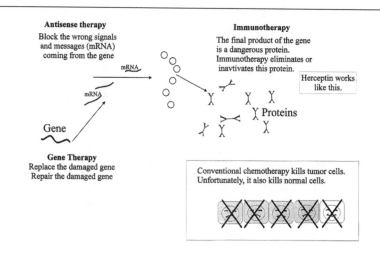

Antisense therapy

Block the wrong signals and messages (mRNA) coming from the gene

Immunotherapy

The final product of the gene is a dangerous protein. Immunotherapy eliminates or inavtivates this protein.

Herceptin works like this.

mRNA

Proteins

Gene

Gene Therapy
Replace the damaged gene
Repair the damaged gene

Conventional chemotherapy kills tumor cells. Unfortunately, it also kills normal cells.

Figure 11.2 (top) Treatment Strategies and
Figure 11.3 (bottom) Future Therapies.

most others)—there have been few breakthroughs. However, there have been many little ones, and the cumulative value of these adds up to better overall care.

As I was revising this book for the last time, The Lancet published a new, exciting study by Professor Peto and his colleagues at Oxford.[25] It looks as if the mortality rates from breast cancer in the U.K. have dropped by over 20 percent in the last ten years. The authors attributed this to a combination of early detection by mammography screening and earlier and better treatment. In particular, they said that the results were due to the use of the estrogen-receptor blocking drug, Tamoxifen. The results in the U.K. were somewhat better than in the U.S., because British doctors began using this drug earlier than their American colleagues. Importantly, this drug is easy to take, is inexpensive, and has relatively few side effects. We can only hope that in the immediate future we will have some more genuine "breakthroughs." Eventually, we will overcome breast cancer. In the meantime, each little step forward is significant.

Appendix: Sensitivity, Specificity, and Predictive Values of Screening Tests

Highly *sensitive* tests detect almost all cases of disease, but they often detect abnormalities in subjects who do not have disease. On the other hand, highly *specific* tests will detect only the disease. The disadvantage of these is that they may miss cases. So it is best to screen with a highly sensitive test, and then confirm the diagnosis with a specific test (e.g., a biopsy).

If someone with disease has a positive test we call this a "True Positive" test. If someone does not have the disease and the test is negative, we call this a "True Negative" test.

	Test	*Disease*
True Positive (TP)	+	+
False Positive (FP)	+	–
False Negative (FN)	–	+
True Negative (TN)	–	–

A positive test can have two disease states, (a) present or (b) absent, and the sensitivity and specificity of the tests are calculated as follows.

	Disease	
Test Result	Present	Absent
Positive	TP	FP
Negative	FN	TN

Sensitivity = TP/(TP+FN) **Specificity** = TN/(FP+TN)

139

Another way for stating these is:

Sensitivity = Number with disease who have a positive test
                          Number with disease

Specificity = Number without disease who have a negative test
                          Number without disease

The value of a diagnostic test depends on factors other than sensitivity and specificity. In particular, a low prevalence of disease influences the likelihood of false positives appearing. Prevalence, in turn, influences "prior probability." So, the rarer a disease is, such as breast cancer in a normal asymptomatic 50-year-old woman, the more specific a test must be, to be clinically useful. "Prior probability" refers to the likelihood of a patient having a disease, based on the statistical prevalence of that disease in a specific population. For example, a 25-year-old healthy male athlete with chest pain would have a prior probability of having significant coronary artery disease of possibly one percent or less. Statistically, the chest pain would almost certainly be due to something other than coronary artery disease. In a 55-year-old male smoker with chest pain, the prior probability of significant coronary artery disease might be greater than 90 percent.

The relationship between sensitivity/specificity of a test and prior probability gives us "predictive values." These are far more useful clinical indicators than sensitivity or specificity on their own. A positive predictive value of a test is the probability that a person with a positive test actually has the disease. A negative predictive value of a test is the probability that a person with a negative test does not have the disease. Predictive values are calculated from the following formulas:

Positive Predictive value =

                    Number with disease and a positive (abnormal) test
                    Number with a positive test

Negative Predictive Value =

                    Number without disease with a negative test
                    Number with a negative test

(Source: SB Hulley et al., Designing clinical research: an epidemiologic approach, Lippincott Williams & Wilkins, 2000, 2nd ed.; D Coogan, G Rose and DJ Barker, Epidemiology for the uninitiated, BMJ Books, 1999, 4th ed.)

Glossary

Acinus: Unit of breast cells responsible for making milk. A collection of acini make up the lobule. Lobular carcinomas arise from here.

Adenine: This is one of the four bases making up the DNA and RNA codes.

ADH: Atypical Ductal Hyperplasia. Its relevance depends on the context in which it is found. Ductal cells show nuclear abnormalities short of malignancy. In needle biopsies this change may be seen beside ductal carcinomas. While it is commonly regarded as a precursor to malignancy, it usually does not progress to cancer.

Adhesion molecule: A chemical that binds cells to each other and also to connective tissue.

AIDS: Acquired Immune Deficiency Syndrome.

Alternative medicine: Methods that use diet, folk remedies, herbal remedies, or various bioelectromagnetic techniques. In general, these are techniques that are unproven regarding their curative value. However, they have been popularized in the lay press and by testimonials from individual patients. Many of them may make the patient feel better and may have a placebo effect.

Amino acid: Small molecules that can link together to form proteins. There are 20 different common amino acids and the way they link to each other and the number of amino acids that are linked together can produce thousands of different proteins with very different properties.

Anemia: Low hemoglobin. Hemoglobin is the oxygen-carrying protein present in the red blood cells. There are many causes. The commonest is iron deficiency.

Angiogenesis: The growth of (new) blood vessels.

Angiogenesis growth factor: A substance secreted by tumors which induces the surrounding tissue to sprout tiny capillaries, also called tumor angiogenesis growth factor (TAF). New blood vessels help tumor cells to metastasize. They also deliver blood with its oxygen and nutrients to the tumor cells.

Antibody: A special type of protein that binds to target antigens. Antibodies are helpful in eliminating bacteria and other foreign microorganisms. They are also produced in response to antigens present in tumor cells. Antibodies are produced by lymphocytes and circulate in the blood and other body fluids. The detection of antibodies against tumor antigens may be helpful in diagnosis or in monitoring cancer patients after treatment.

Antigen: A molecule, usually a protein, which has the ability to stimulate lymphocytes to produce antibodies.

Apoptosis: A form of cell death characterized by shrinkage of the cell and its contents. The apoptotic cell is eliminated by macrophages. Apoptosis is a normal physiological process by which cells are eliminated after they have lived their normal life cycle. The process is controlled by a number of genes; the best known is the bcl 2 oncogene. In many cancers the tumor cells are not eliminated, but persist indefinitely.

Ataxia: Loss of balance due to poor coordination. This can result from a large number of disorders affecting the brain or inner ear.

Ataxia-telangiectasia: A rare genetic disorder characterized by ataxia and immune deficiency. Patients with ataxia-telangiectasia are more prone to breast cancer. The gene responsible for this condition has been recently identified and characterized.

Axilla: The armpit. It contains fat, blood vessels, nerves, and lymph nodes. These lymph nodes are frequently sampled or removed during the surgery for breast cancer. Examination of the lymph nodes helps to determine the stage of the tumor (how far it has spread).

Base: The chemicals making up the coding region of the DNA molecule are called bases. These are adenine, guanine, cytosine, and thymine.

Base pair: The combination of two bases within the DNA molecule. A always combines with T, and C with G.

Basement membrane: A protein membrane that separates epithelium from underlying connective tissue. Basement membrane also separates blood vessel endothelial cells from the underlying muscle cells. It provides a temporary barrier to the growth of cancer in epithelial tissues. Cancer confined to cells above the basement membrane is called carcinoma in situ and cannot metastasize until it has broken through the basement membrane.

Bcl 2 oncogene: This is a gene that codes for apoptosis. In some low-grade cancers cell proliferation can be less than normal tissue. However, due to activity of the bcl 2 oncogene tumor cells persist indefinitely. They accumulate and cause the tumor to grow.

Benign tumor: Benign neoplasm. This is a new growth or a tumor which does not invade and destroy normal tissues, or metastasize. It can be composed of epithelial tissue or stroma (such as muscle). However, it can cause symptoms by local pressure on surrounding tissues. For example, in the uterus it may cause bleeding from the surface of the endometrium. If they arise in an endocrine gland sometimes benign tumors are functionally active. They may produce the same hormone as the tissue from which they arise. Benign tumors rarely become malignant. However, some, such as adenomas or polyps in the intestine, may evolve into malignancy over a period of many years. The most common breast tumor is the fibroadenoma. It is benign.

Biopsy: Removal of a piece of tissue for microscopic examination. This may be a tiny fragment (less than 1 mm) removed through a needle or it may be a large excision biopsy. Many biopsies remove just a sample of tissue 2 to 3 mm in size for initial diagnostic purposes. In addition to making a diagnosis, the pathologist can often grade the tumor on the basis of the biopsy. Sometimes, for example with a breast lump, the biopsy procedure may be therapeutic (excision biopsy) as the entire lesion may be removed by the biopsy.

Bone marrow: Soft spongy tissue residing within the bone marrow spaces. The cells comprising this tissue give rise to circulating blood cells—red blood cells, white blood cells and platelets.

Bone Marrow Transplant (BMT): Some patients benefit from extra high dose chemotherapy. Under normal circumstances such chemotherapy would wipe out the patient's marrow completely and leave them prone to overwhelming infection with a high risk of death. Bone marrow transplantation can protect such patients. The bone marrow comes either from the donor herself or from someone with closely related transplantation genes (usually someone from the same family).

Brachytherapy: A form of radiation therapy whereby radioactive particles are embedded directly into the tissue (as distinct from external beam radiation).

BRCA1: Approximately ten percent of breast cancers are familial and are due to hereditary genetic mutations. Those that have been identified to date are mostly in the genes known as BRCA1and BRCA2. Women with mutations in these genes have a high incidence of breast cancer and also ovarian cancer. The precise function of BRCA1 and BRCA2 under normal circumstances is not known.

BRCA2: Like BRCA1, mutations in this gene are responsible for many of the familial breast and ovarian cancers.

Breast-conserving surgery: Removal of cancer leaving the uninvolved breast intact. More and more, this is becoming an alternative to mastectomy.

Cancer: Common term to include any form of malignancy.

Carcinogen: Common term used to describe anything that can cause cancer.

Carcinoma: A malignant tumor arising from epithelial tissue. Most adult cancers are carcinomas.

Carcinoma in situ: The early phase of malignant epithelial tumors, which is confined above a basement membrane. Carcinoma in situ cannot metastasize until it has transformed into an invasive carcinoma and has penetrated the basement membrane. Carcinoma in situ is commonly seen in the skin, breast, cervix and intestine.

Case control study: A form of scientific investigation where a group of patients with a certain medical problem, for example, breast cancer, is compared to a group of people who do not have that medical problem. Two groups are similar in age (and sex) and many other variables. They are studied to determine what factors (such as cigarette smoking, living in a certain location, etc.) might be linked with the disease. This is a form of epidemiological study.

Cell: The smallest completely independent structure of a tissue or organ. It is the basic functional unit of all living tissue. Each cell is composed of an outer cell membrane and an inner bag of fluid, enzymes and proteins. Within this the nucleus exists as a separate membrane-bound structure. Chromosomes and genetic material are contained within the nucleus. Tiny organelles are structures present in the cytoplasm and these are responsible for directing the cell's metabolism.

Cell cycle: Most cells grow, divide, and form new daughter cells. This process of cell proliferation is controlled by a large number of genes and the process has different phases known as G0, G1, S, G2, and M. (See other names below.) Some cells have a rapid cell cycle such as bone marrow cells, cells lining the skin, and cells lining the intestine. Some cells such as neurons do not divide. Other cells proliferate when injured or stimulated. Tumor cells have very abnormal cell cycles.

Chemotherapy: Treatment for cancer that involves primarily the use of drugs (as distinct from surgery and radiation therapy).

Chromosome: Each cell contains 46 chromosomes. Each chromosome consists of complex, compactly folded strands of DNA. The DNA is wound around a protein core. Half of the genetic material is derived from each parent. When a cell divides its chromosomes split and reduplicate, with an equal amount of DNA going into each of the daughter cells.

Clinical trial: A scientific investigation carried out under rigorous conditions to compare the value and complications of one particular type of treatment with another. Often neither the doctors nor the patients know which treatment they are receiving (double blind trial).

Clone: A group of cells, all derived from one single cell. Most cancers are thought to be monoclonal in origin. However, during their growth, tumors frequently have subclones with different characteristics and biological advantages.

Cohort study: A scientific epidemiological study in which a large population (possibly 100,000) are questioned in detail about their habits and their environment. The population is then followed for a number of years or decades to see who gets sick and who doesn't. Researchers analyze the data and try to identify what factors might account for the difference between those who get sick and those who don't.

Collagen: Common type of connective tissue protein that acts as a scaffolding for cells in almost all organs, including the breast. It is also a major component of basement membranes, blood vessels, and scars. When there is an increased amount in the breast it can cause a lump (as in fibrocystic change).

Computerized image analysis: A process whereby microscopic and other images are read and analyzed by computers. The analysis can be completely automated or it may allow an observer to interact in decision-making tasks. Computerized image analyses are commonly used in research on tissues and cells. They can also be used in diagnostic cytology.

Connective tissue: Connective tissue is a loose substance composed of cells, water, proteins (including collagen), and other chemicals that surround and bind together muscles, nerves, blood vessels, and all tissues in all organs. It is also known as stroma.

Cowden's syndrome: A genetic disorder characterized by a combination of intestinal polyps and benign tumors of the skin and uterus. These patients have an increased risk for breast cancer.

Cyst: A lump or bump composed of a collection of fluid with a surrounding thin wall. It is benign.

Cytologist: Medical technologist, specially trained to identify malignant and pre-malignant changes in cytology preparations, such as cervical cytology smears.

Cytology: The microscopic study of cellular abnormalities in preparations that were made by smearing cells onto a glass slide. It differs from histology in that entire cells or groups of cells are examined but little or no tissue architecture is present. In contrast, histology preparations show microarchitecture. Because histology preparations show cells growing in relation to each other and also in relationship to basement membrane and stroma, histologic appearances tend to be more definitive than cytology.

Cytosine: One of the four bases making up the DNA code (also see adenine, thymine, and guanine).

DCIS: See Ductal carcinoma in situ.

Deoxyribose: The sugar molecule that makes up the outer structure of the DNA helix.

Diagnostic cytology: The microscopic study of cells removed from a visible abnormality. If the lesion is deep within the body it may be localized using radiological procedures. In such circumstances a fine needle is introduced into the abnormality and cells are aspirated. Screening cytology is the term used to describe the examination of cells that are removed from a normal person, as part of a screening procedure rather than directly from a visible lesion. Cervical cytology, where the doctor removes cells randomly from the surface of the cervix, is a typical examination of screening cytology.

Differentiation: The process whereby normal cells and tissue mature toward their final appearance, e.g., brain, heart, liver. In cancer, it refers to the process whereby the tumor tissue tries to simulate as close as possible the tissue from which it arose. The term well-differentiated means the tumor closely resembles normal tissue. Poorly differentiated tumors do not bear a close resemblance to the tissue they originated from. The term undifferentiated refers to a tumor with a primitive embryonic appearance bearing no resemblance to any normal tissue.

Digital mammography: Use of digital images (computer generated) instead of conventional x-ray images. Up to now the quality of such images has been inferior to those obtained by conventional x-ray film. Within the next few years it is expected that this form of digital radiography will rival the current methodology in terms of quality, cost and practicality.

DNA: Deoxyribonucleic acid, a molecule with a double helix configuration responsible for storing and passing on genetic information. All genes are made from DNA.

DNA vaccine: New form of immunotherapy that uses specific gene fragments that code for specific antigens. These vaccines have not yet found their place in cancer therapy. However, there is much research in this area.

Ductal carcinoma: The most common type of breast cancer. It may be in situ, where it is confined to the epithelium lining the breast ducts (ductal carcinoma in situ). More commonly it is invasive and called invasive ductal carcinoma.

Ductal carcinoma in situ (DCIS): Malignant cells confined within lumen of ducts. These cells cannot metastasize until they have invaded through the duct wall into the surrounding stroma.

Endoglin and endosialin: Molecules in the endothelial cells lining blood vessels in tumors. These may prove to be useful targets for new treatments directed at such blood vessels. If researchers can destroy these vessels, they will starve the tumor of oxygen and nutrition. In the process the tumor will be destroyed.

Enzyme: A protein that speeds up chemical reactions in tissues. Enzymes may act within the cell to speed up the synthesis of molecules. However, enzymes are also secreted from the cancer cell into their surrounding environment where they may help the cancer to invade and destroy tissue and spread.

Epidemiology: The scientific study of how disease affects large populations, rather than individuals. It uses biostatistics as its main tool to investigate the association between illness and possible causes. By identifying associations, epidemiologists may provide clues about the cause of a specific disease. However, it does not provide proof. Methods other than observation and association are required for proof of causation. Epidemiological studies are classified as descriptive or analytic. Descriptive studies determine the nature of the population affected with a specific disease, taking into account such factors as age, sex, ethnic origin, and occupation. Descriptive studies may identify new diseases or suggest a previously unrecognized association between a risk factor and a disease. Analytic studies test the conclusions drawn from descriptive surveys, or from laboratory observations. Case control studies and cohort studies (see above) are forms of epidemiological analytic studies. The results of epidemiological studies may be used to plan new health services, such as cancer screening, or to evaluate the overall health of a given population.

Epithelial cell: Epithelial cells line the inside of most organs, including the breast. Here, they line the ducts and lobules. A collection of lining epithelial cells is called epithelium.

Epithelium: The covering or lining of organs. For example, the outer layer of the skin and the inner layers of lungs, intestinal tract, urinary tract, uterus and vagina, blood vessels and various ducts are all lined by epithelium.

False negative diagnosis: This is when a patient is diagnosed as not having a particular disease, when in reality the patient has the disease. This is a relatively rare occurrence when combinations of methods or tests are used before arriving at a final diagnosis. However, it is not uncommon for a single test to have a false negative result. Sometimes, especially in the early stages of the disease, some tests may be positive and some tests may be negative and the physician ends up with an inconclusive result. The diagnostic process is put on temporary hold. After a period of time (often months) the tests are repeated. Usually the correct diagnosis becomes apparent after a period of time and observation.

False positive diagnosis: This occurs when a patient is diagnosed as having a particular disease, when in reality she does not have the disease. This is even less common than a false negative diagnosis.

Familial Adenomatosis Polyposis (FAP): A hereditary condition, characterized by the presence of dozens to thousands of polyps throughout the colon. These are premalignant and due to a genetic mutation on chromosome 5. Colectomy is the treatment of choice and prevents the onset of cancer.

Fat necrosis: Damage to the fat cells in the breast. This causes thickening and hardening of tissue and often produces an irregular lump that can be confused clinically and mammographically with cancer.

Fibroadenoma: A benign tumor of the breast composed of a mixture of epithelium and connective tissue.

Fibrocystic disease (change): A benign condition of the breast characterized by the presence of cysts, increased glandular proliferation and increased fibrous tissue. Its importance is that it produces a lump that must be distinguished from cancer. Minor degrees of fibrocystic change are so common as to be regarded as a variation of normal. The term "fibrocystic disease" is gradually disappearing from medical terminology and it is being replaced by "fibrocystic change."

Fibrous tissue: Dense connective tissue composed of collagen and other similar proteins, without epithelial components.

Fine Needle Aspiration (FNA) cytology: A technique for removing tiny numbers of cells through a fine bore needle. Its main advantage is that it can get a sample of the cells from deeply located lesions without surgery. A very fine needle is inserted into the lesion. If the lesion is superficial or palpable the procedure can be carried out by a surgeon, pathologist, or a physician trained to carry out the technique. If the lesion is deep seated within the lung, pancreas, or some other internal organ, the procedure is usually carried out by a radiologist under CT (computerized tomography) or ultrasound guidance. The disadvantage of the technique is that it has a moderately high false negative result (depending on the lesion being sampled) and the specimen provided is, in general, inferior to a tissue biopsy. However, it is often a safe, efficient and cost effective method of obtaining a rapid diagnosis.

Five-year survival: This term is commonly used to evaluate response to treatment and prognosis. Usually patients who survive for five years, with no evidence of recurrent disease, are cured. However, depending on the particular cancer, some tumors recur even after five years. The term does not equate with absolute cure.

FNA: See fine needle aspiration cytology.

G0: The resting phase of the cell cycle.

G1: The first gap phase of the cell cycle.

G2: The second gap phase of the cell cycle. Various enzymes and gene regulators accumulate in preparation for cell division.

Gene: Genes are those fragments of DNA that code for a specific chemical product (e.g., a protein) or human characteristic.

Gene chip: New powerful technology that combines molecular biology and computer technology to identify DNA mutations and signals coming from genes.

Gene therapy: A form of treatment in which a defective gene can be repaired or replaced by a normal gene. This form of therapy for cancer is still at the experimental stage.

Grade: The degree of malignancy as determined by microscopic examination. There are many different grading systems. However, most cancers can be divided into low, intermediate, and high grades. In general, low-grade tumors grow slowly and are biologically less aggressive than high grade tumors. They tend to be more amenable to surgical removal, metastasize later, and do not respond well to chemotherapy. There are many exceptions to these generalizations.

Growth receptor: A protein that sits somewhere in a cell (often on the outer membrane) and accepts specific molecules. The receptor then sends a signal to induce the cell to grow. In many cancers, there are too many receptors present.

Guanine: One of the four bases that make up the DNA code.

Halsted's operation: Radical mastectomy. This removes the breast, underlying muscle, and lymph nodes in the axilla—rarely done today.

HeLa tumor cells: Immortalized tumor cells used for research in laboratories throughout the world.

Helix: A coiled, spiral-like structure found in many molecules, including DNA.

HER-2/neu: A growth promoting gene (oncogene) that functions by producing excess growth receptors. This gene is overactive in many breast cancers.

Herceptin: A monoclonal antibody drug used to block the action of HER-2/neu.

Hereditary: A condition or characteristic inherited from ones' parents or grandparents.

Histopathology: The microscopic study of disease.

Hormone: This is a chemical released from one tissue that passes into circulation and exerts its influence on another distant tissue. Typical examples are insulin, growth hormone, epinephrine, and estrogen.

Hyperplasia: An increase in the number of cells in any tissue. In the breast, the epithelial cells lining the ducts often show hyperplasia in fibrocystic disease. It is not usually premalignant.

Immune cells: Cells responsible for immunological reactions. These are T or B cells (lymphocytes). Macrophages also play a role in the immunological system by processing information for the T and B cells.

Immunotherapy: A form of therapy designed to enhance the body's immune system against disease. In relation to cancer, it attempts to trick immune cells into thinking that cancer cells are foreign cells and should be rejected.

LCIS: See lobular carcinoma in situ.

Li-Fraumeni syndrome: A rare disorder characterized by the presence of many different cancers in the same individual. It is due to an inherited mutation of the p53 gene.

Lobular carcinoma: A type of breast cancer, arising from the lobular epithelium. Infiltrating lobular carcinoma in one of the two more common breast cancers (the other is infiltrating ductal carcinoma).

Lobular carcinoma in situ (LCIS): Tissue change confined to lobules that carries an increased risk for subsequent breast cancer. It is also known as lobular neoplasia in situ.

Local invasion: This has the same meaning as local spread.

Local spread: Spread to adjacent tissues. For example, cancer of the thyroid gland spreads through the thyroid into the surrounding connective tissue in the neck.

Lumpectomy: A term commonly applied to a surgical procedure to remove a tumor with minimal surrounding normal tissue. Breast cancers are frequently removed by lumpectomy.

Lymph nodes: Small collections of lymphocytes and macrophages (bound together in packages, surrounded by a thin layer of connective tissue). Lymphatic channels lead into and out from each lymph node. There are hundreds of lymph nodes scattered throughout the body. They are the main tissues of the immune system. Within lymph nodes, lymphocytes proliferate in response to an immunological insult or stimulus.

Lymphatics: These are the tiny thread-like channels carrying fluid into, and from, lymph nodes. Within the lymphatic fluid, lymphocytes travel to and from lymph nodes. Lymphatics and their lymph nodes monitor every tissue in the body.

Lymphocyte: The cells controlling the immune system. They are classified as T lymphocytes and B lymphocytes. Lymphatic and lymphoblastic leukemias arise from lymphocytes as do non–Hodgkin's lymphomas.

M phase: The mitotic phase of the cell cycle during which cells divide to form two daughter cells.

Macrophage: An immune cell responsible for destruction of injurious foreign material and infections. It plays a major role in modifying and preparing molecules so that other immune cells can recognize and destroy "foreign" cells, including tumor cells.

Malignant lymphoma: A malignant tumor arising from lymphoid tissue in lymph nodes and other tissues. Lymphomas are classified into two main groups—non–Hodgkin's lymphomas and Hodgkin's disease.

Mammography: A special x-ray of the breasts, used to identify and localize breast cancer. Its main advantage is that it can detect carcinoma in situ (pre-cancer) or very small infiltrating carcinomas—too small to be clinically palpable.

Mastectomy: Surgical removal of the breast. A simple mastectomy removes the breast and overlying skin but no underlying deep tissues. A radical mastectomy removes the breast with underlying muscle, connective tissue and axillary contents. Radical mastectomies are rarely performed now, as less radical surgical procedures achieve the same effect and are less mutilating.

MDM2: An oncogene conferring aggressive behavior characteristics on tumor cells.

Medline: An electronic database containing the names of all published articles in the medical literature since the mid–1960s, including a summary of most articles.

Metastases: Spread of tumor from one site to another. Breast cancer commonly metastasizes to lymph nodes, liver, lungs, bone, and brain.

Micrometastases: Metastases consisting of one or a few cells. They may be too small to be detected by routine light microscopy. However, more sensitive molecular biology techniques can detect may different forms of micrometastases. The clinical significance of micrometastases is not yet clear. As might be expected, some recent studies show that they reduce survival time.

Mismatch repair gene: Each cell has a set of genes whose function is to repair minor damage to the DNA molecule. Certain individuals have mutations in these repair genes. Minor degrees of DNA damage accumulate with repeated cell divisions and eventually cancer follows. Mutated mismatch repair genes are found most commonly in patients with hereditary non-polyposis colon cancer.

Mitosis: The process by which a cell splits and divides into two other cells. Each of the new cells has the same genetic material as the original cell.

Molecular biology techniques: Techniques that employ the isolation and analysis of DNA or RNA.

Monoclonal: Arising from one cell. All cells in the monoclonal group or tumor show similar characteristics to the cell from which they arose.

mRNA: Messenger RNA. This molecule carries signals from the DNA in the nucleus to the ribosomes within the cytoplasm. In the ribosomes the signals are translated into amino acids and proteins.

Mucinous (colloid) carcinoma: A special type of invasive ductal carcinoma that usually is low grade and has a good prognosis. It gets its name from the fact that the tumor cells secrete large quantities of mucin (a combination of proteins, water, and carbohydrate-rich material).

Mutation: Any structural alteration of a gene that results in the wrong message being sent to the cytoplasm and subsequently a defective protein or function. Mutations can be acquired or inherited. Common inherited disorders are sickle cell anemia, cystic fibrosis and muscular dystrophy.

Myoepithelial cell: Myoepithelial cells surround the epithelial cells in ducts and acini (lobules). They are contractile cells and help move milk along the ducts toward the nipple.

NCI: National Cancer Institute. This is a subdivision of the National Institutes of Health (NIH) and is responsible for most government-sponsored cancer research funding in the U.S.

NIH: National Institutes of Health.

NM23: A gene whose function is not fully understood. It may play a role in preventing metastases.

Nodes: Short for lymph nodes or lymph glands.

Nuclear atypia: The dysplastic abnormal nuclei seen in cancer and pre-malignancy.

Nucleus: Membrane-bound structure in the center of the cell. It consists of proteins and water and contains the cells' chromosomes and their genes. Sometimes benign conditions can cause atypical nuclei and mimic dysplastic changes.

OAM: Office of Alternative Medicine.

Occupational cancers: Cancers that have been associated with specific occupations such as shipbuilding (asbestos-related mesothelioma), uranium mining, dye manufacture, or the manufacture of polyvinylchloride.

Oncogene: Oncogenes are present in normal cells and contribute to the regulation of cell growth. In cancer they may be amplified or over-active and drive the tumor cell to proliferate rapidly and out of control.

Oncologist: Medically qualified doctor who specializes in treating cancer patients.

Organ: This term is used for any fully formed tissue in the body such as heart, lung, brain, or kidney.

p53 gene: This oncogene is responsible for controlling many aspects of the cell cycle and also contributes to the control of apoptosis. It is mutated in over 50 percent of all cancers.

Palliative treatment: Treatment aimed at alleviating pain and ensuring that the patient can live in relative comfort. It does not attempt to eradicate cancer completely.

Pap smear test: The Pap tested is named after Dr. Papanicolaou who first used cytology for diagnosing cancer and precancer. The Pap smear or Pap test refers to the microscopic examination of cells taken from the surface of the cervix.

Pathologist: A medically qualified doctor who specializes in the examination of tissue, blood, fluid, or secretions for diagnostic purposes. The term is most commonly used to describe histopathologists who microscopically examine biopsies and surgically removed tissue. They are also known as surgical pathologists. They diagnose, grade, and stage cancer.

PCR: Polymerase chain reaction. A molecular biology technique for amplifying tiny fragments of DNA or RNA. After amplification the DNA or RNA can then be analyzed.

Peptide: A group of amino acids linked together. Amino acids and peptides are assembled to form proteins.

Pharmacologist: Scientist who studies the mechanisms and effects of chemical compounds (drugs).

Pituitary gland: A pea-sized gland at the base of the brain that secretes a variety of hormones. These control the activity of the thyroid, the adrenal glands, the ovaries, the testes and body growth. It also produces a hormone called prolactin which controls milk secretion by the breast epithelial cells in the acinus/lobule.

Polyclonal: Benign tumors are due to growth of cells derived from many different cells. In contrast, most cancers arise from the continued growth of a single cell. Proliferation from many different cells is referred to as polyclonal, whereas proliferation from a single cell is termed monoclonal.

Poorly differentiated: Tumors that bear little resemblance to the original tissue from which they arose are classified as poorly differentiated. In general, poorly differentiated tumors are aggressive. (Also see well differentiated.)

Precancer: Cellular changes that precede cancer. A typical example is dysplasia of the cervical epithelium. Sometimes dysplastic changes revert back to normal. Sometimes they progress to invasive cancer.

Premalignant: Conditions that may progress to cancer over a long time, such as chronic ulcers, Barrett's esophagus, or colonic polyps. In the breast, ADH is often regarded as a premalignant lesion.

Primary tumor: The first or original tumor. The term is used to distinguish the primary tumor from metastatic tumors, which are sometimes referred to as secondaries. Theoretically, each organ in the body can be the site of either primary or secondary (metastatic) tumors. Occasionally the distinction between primary tumor and metastatic tumor may be difficult (for example, in the ovary). A patient may have more than one primary tumor.

Prognosis: The long-term outlook for a patient with disease. For cancer patients it is commonly measured as five-year survival (see above).

Promoter: In classical experimental carcinogenesis, in order to produce a malignancy it was necessary to use two sets of chemicals. The first was called an initiator, and this started the carcinogenic process but required the presence of a second chemical, called a promoter, to finish the process of cancer formation. In clinical practice it is not known how often this experimental concept is recapitulated. However, it is clear that carcinogenic agents frequently assist each other and are referred to as co-factors. For example, asbestos causes malignant mesothelioma (a malignancy of the lining of the lung) and cigarette smoking causes lung cancer arising from the bronchi. Cigarette smokers who are also exposed to asbestos have a much greater risk for developing primary lung cancer than those exposed to cigarette smoke only.

Promoter gene: A gene that influences or controls another gene. Promoter genes play an important role in switching on or switching off those genes responsible for cell proliferation.

Radiation therapy: One form of cancer treatment that may be used alone or in combination with surgery and chemotherapy. Some tumors are very radiosensitive and in certain circumstances radiation therapy can achieve the same result as surgery. However, like surgery, it is confined to localized treatment of the primary tumor and its immediately adjacent tissues. It may also be helpful as a palliative procedure for reducing tumor bulk or pain, for example, with metastases to the spine.

Radical lymph node dissection: Some cancers spread to draining lymph nodes and remain there for a long time, before metastasizing widely. Under such circumstances radical removal of an entire group of lymph nodes may be curative. A common example is cancer of the larynx (voice box) that has spread to the lymph nodes in the neck. Radical dissection of lymph nodes in the neck may prevent subsequent spread. However, in breast cancer, radical removal of axillary lymph nodes does not improve the prognosis.

Radioresistant: The term refers to tumors that do not respond to radiation treatment.

Radiosensitive: For some tissues and tumors, radiation is highly lethal. Such tumors are radiosensitive.

Radiotherapist: A medically qualified doctor who treats patients with radiation therapy.

Radiotherapy (Radiation therapy): This may be administered on its own or in combination with surgery or chemotherapy. The radiation dose may be administered by external beam radiation or by implantation of radioactive materials into the tumor. It may also be delivered (rarely) by administration of isotopes that selectively bind to tumor tissue.

Reticuloendothelial system: Part of the immune system. Macrophages and other cells, like macrophages, are scattered throughout the body and collectively are called the reticuloendothelial system.

Ribosome: Thousands of tiny organelles called ribosomes reside in the cytoplasm of each cell. The ribosome is responsible for converting the message from DNA into amino acids and proteins. Cells that manufacture abundant protein are particularly rich in ribosomes.

Risk ratio: A term used by epidemiologists to quantify the risk of disease associated with a particular occupation, event, drug, or any other variable. The measurement is made in comparison to what would happen if the variable were absent.

RNA: Ribonucleic acid. During the course of protein synthesis an instruction is transferred from the DNA in the nucleus to the ribosomes in the cytoplasm through a messenger molecule made from RNA. This is called messenger RNA or mRNA. There are other forms of RNA also present in the cell.

S phase: The phase during the cell cycle in which DNA is synthesized from existing DNA.

Screening cytology: Microscopic examination of cells in an attempt to detect premalignant changes. Screening cytology is carried out particularly in the prevention of cervical cancer.

SEER: The Surveillance, Epidemiology and End Results program of the National Cancer Institute (NCI) in Washington. This is one of the organizations that provides population-based cancer statistics in the U.S.

Segmentectomy: Surgical term for removal of a breast segment.

Sporadic: When used in the context of cancer it refers to tumors that occur randomly with no hereditary background.

Stage: See tumor stage.

Stem cell transplant: Bone marrow and blood cells come from stem cells. High dose chemotherapy destroys the bone marrow. It is now possible to harvest stem cells from peripheral blood, and this can be done before chemotherapy. Stem cells are returned to the patient's blood after chemotherapy, by intravenous infusion. They repopulate the bone marrow and change (differentiate) into normal marrow and blood cells. Stem cell transplantation has revolutionized the treatment of certain malignancies, such as leukemia and lymphoma. Despite early promise, it has not proven very useful in breast cancer.

Stroma: See connective tissue.

Suicide genes: A popular term used for those genes controlling the process of apoptosis. (Also see apoptosis.)

Tamoxifen: An antihormone drug used in the treatment of breast cancer. It is particularly useful for tumors that are rich in estrogen receptors. Estrogens often enhance breast cancer growth and in order to do this they must bind to estrogen receptors present in breast cancer cells. Tamoxifen blocks the binding of estrogen to its receptor and thus removes the estrogen growth effect.

Telomerase: An enzyme that maintains telomere length. Cancer cells have active telomerase that contributes to tumor cell immortality.

Telomere: Segments of chromosomal ends that act as molecular clocks. Each time a cell divides it loses pieces of its telomeres. At some critical level of shortening normal cells can no longer divide. Cancer cells have long telomeres due to the activity of telomerase.

Thymine: One of the DNA bases used to form the genetic code.

Tissue: Each organ in the body is made up of thousands of cells that are bound together into different layers, referred to as tissue. It is a general term used for layers of cells in any organ in the body.

Tumor stage: This refers to the extent a tumor has spread from its original site. There are many different staging systems used; however, they are all based on similar principles. For convenience we can think of tumor spread as having three major steps. Stage I is when the tumor is confined to the tissue from which it has arisen. Stage II refers to tumor that has spread to draining lymph nodes, and Stage III refers to tumor that has spread to distal organs such as liver or bone marrow. Often those stages have subdivisions, or frequently a four-stage system rather than a three-stage system is used.

Tumor suppressor gene: A gene whose function is to slow down a particular activity, such as cell growth.

Tumor type: The histopathologic classification, e.g., ductal carcinoma, lobular carcinoma.

Tumorigenesis: A general term used to describe the development and progression of cancer.

Ultrasound examination: An imaging technique using ultrasound waves to outline the size, shape, and consistency of internal organs. Its most common use is in assessing the development of a fetus in utero. However, many abdominal organs can be visualized very well using ultrasound. Its main advantages are that it is non-invasive and does not use any ionizing radiation (x-rays). It is very reliable in distinguishing cystic from solid tumors or tumor-like masses.

Undifferentiated: An undifferentiated tumor is one that shows no resemblance to the tissue from which it has arisen. It is a stage beyond "poorly differentiated." Most undifferentiated malignant tumors, no matter where they have arisen, tend to resemble each other, microscopically.

Well differentiated: Having a microscopic appearance very similar to normal tissue.

Wilms' tumor: A form of kidney cancer in infants and children. Most are sporadic. However, a small percentage is hereditary.

Notes

1. The Scourge of Breast Cancer and the Scope of the Problem

1. Devesa SS, Blot WJ, Stone BJ, Miller BA, Tarone RE, Fraumeni JF, Jr. Recent cancer trends in the United States. Journal of the National Cancer Institute 1995; 87:175–182.

2. Chu KC, Tarone RE, Kessler LG, Ries LA, Hankey BF, Miller BA et al. Recent trends in U.S. breast cancer incidence, survival, and mortality rates. Journal of the National Cancer Institute 1996; 88(21):1571–1579.

3. Berg JW, Hutter RV. Breast cancer. Cancer 1995; 75(1 Suppl): 257–269.

4. SEER data. (1999). http://www.seer.ims.nci.nih.gov/

5. American Cancer Society. (1999). http://www.cancer.org/statistics/

6. Bunker JP, Houghton J, Baum M. Putting the risk of breast cancer in perspective. British Medical Journal 1998; 317(7168):1307–1309.

7. Phillips KA, Glendon G, Knight JA. Putting the risk of breast cancer in perspective. New England Journal of Medicine 1999; 340(2):141–144.

8. Program to download to assess absolute from relative risk (Vanderbilt Medical Center, Nashville, TN). (1999). http://www.mc.vanderbilt.edu/prevmed/absrisk.htm

9. Blumenthal D. Health care reform at the close of the 20th century. New England Journal of Medicine 1999; 340(24):1916–1920.

10. Holland JC. Cancer's psychological challenges. Scientific American 1996; 275:122–125.

11. Roberts FD, Newcomb PA, Trentham-Dietz A, Storer BE. Self-reported stress and risk of breast cancer. Cancer 1996; 77(6):1089–1093.

12. Oncolink web site. University of Pennsylvania Cancer Center. (1999). http://oncolink.upenn.edu/

13. Muurinen JM. The economics of informal care. Labor market effects in the National Hospice Study. Medical Care 1986; 24(11):1007–1017.

14. Oncolink cancer economics web site. (1999). http://www.oncolink.upenn.edu/pdq_html/cites/10/10320.html

15. Chevarley F, White E. Recent trends in breast cancer mortality among white and black U.S. women. American Journal of Public Health 1997; 87(5):775–781.

16. Garne JP, Aspegren K, Balldin G, Ranstam J. Increasing incidence of and declining mortality from breast carcinoma. Trends in Malmo, Sweden, 1961–1992. Cancer 1997; 79(1):69–74.

17. Gross CP, Anderson GF, Powe NR. The relation between funding by the National Institutes of Health and the burden of disease. New England Journal of Medicine 1999; 340(24):1881–1887.

18. Varmus H. Evaluating the burden of disease and spending the research dollars of the National Institutes of Health. New England Journal of Medicine 1999; 340(24):1914–1915.

2. What Causes Breast Cancer?

1. Bittner JJ. Milk-influence of breast tumors in mice. Science 1942; 95:462–463.

2. Bittner JJ. Some possible effects of nursing on mammary gland tumor incidence in mice. Science 1936; 84:162–163.

3. Bailar JC, Smith EM. Progress against cancer? New England Journal of Medicine 1986; 314:1226–1232.

4. Bailar JC, Gornik HL. Cancer undefeated. New England Journal of Medicine 1997; 336(22):1569–1574.

5. Taubes G. Epidemiology faces its limits. Science 1995; 269(5221):164–169.

6. Petrakis NL. Historic milestones in cancer epidemiology. Seminars in Oncology 1979; 6(4):433–444.

7. Editorial. Tobacco money and medical research. Nature Medicine 1999; 5(2):125.

8. Selikoff IJ, Churg J, Hammond EC. Landmark article April 6, 1964: Asbestos exposure and neoplasia. Journal of The American Medical Association 1984; 252(1):91–95.

9. Selikoff IJ, Churg J, Hammond EC. Relation between exposure to asbestos and mesothelioma. New England Journal of Medicine 1999; 272:560–565.

10. Coffey DS. Self-organization, complexity and chaos: The new biology for medicine. Nature Medicine 1998; 4(8):882–885.

11. Stewart I. Does God play dice? The mathematics of chaos. Blackwell, 1999.

12. DeVita VT, Rosenberg SA, Hellman S. Cancer: principles and practice of oncology. 5 ed. Philadelphia: Lippincott Williams & Wilkins, 1997.

13. Editorial. Pill scares and public responsibility. The Lancet 1996; 347:1707.

14. Wise J. Hormone replacement therapy increases risk of breast cancer. British Medical Journal 1997; 967–972.

15. Harding C, Knox WF, Faragher EB, Baildam A, Bundred NJ. Hormone replacement therapy and tumour grade in breast cancer: prospective study in screening unit. British Medical Journal 1996; 312(7047):1646–1647.

16. Grodstein F, Stampfer MJ, Colditz GA, Willett WC, Manson JE, Joffe M et al. Postmenopausal hormone therapy and mortality. New England Journal of Medicine 1997; 336(25):1769–1775.

17. Mckinney K. Use of hormone replacement therapy. Evidence on risk of breast cancer associated with hormone replacement therapy is still inconclusive. British Medical Journal 1996; 313(7058):686.

18. Collaborative group on hormonal factors in breast cancer. Coordinator V Beral. Breast cancer and hormone replacement therapy: collaborative reanalysis of data from 51 epidemiological studies of 52,705 women with breast cancer and 108,411 women without breast cancer. The Lancet 1997; 350:1047–1059.

19. Colditz GA, Hankinson SE, Hunter DJ, Willett WC, Manson JE, Stampfer MJ et al. The use of estrogens and progestins and the risk of breast cancer in postmenopausal women. New England Journal of Medicine 1995; 332(24):1589–1593.

20. Enger SM, Ross RK, Henderson B, Bernstein L. Breastfeeding history, pregnancy experience and risk of breast cancer. British Journal of Cancer 1997; 76(1):118–123.

21. Newcomb PA, Storer BE, Longnecker MP, Mittendorf R, Greenberg ER, Clapp RW et al. Lactation and a reduced risk of premenopausal breast cancer. New England Journal of Medicine 1994; 330(2):81–87.

22. Michels KB, Willett WC, Rosner BA, Manson JE, Hunter DJ, Colditz GA et al. Prospective assessment of breastfeeding and breast cancer incidence among 89,887 women. The Lancet 1996; 347(8999):431–436.

23. Dupont WD, Page DL. Risk factors for breast cancer in women with proliferative breast disease. New England Journal of Medicine 1985; 312(3):146–151.

24. Fitzgibbons PL, Henson DE, Hutter RV. Benign breast changes and the risk for subsequent breast cancer: an update of the 1985 consensus statement. Cancer Committee of the College of American Pathologists. Archives of Pathology and Laboratory Medicine 1998; 122(12):1053–1055.

25. McDivitt RW, Stevens JA, Lee NC, Wingo PA, Rubin GL, Gersell D. Histologic types of benign breast disease and the risk for breast cancer. The Cancer and Steroid Hormone Study Group. Cancer 1992; 69(6):1408–1414.

26. Michels KB, Willett WC. Does induced or spontaneous abortion affect the risk of breast cancer? Epidemiology 1996; 7(5):521–528.

27. Melbye M, Wohlfahrt J, Olsen JH, Frisch M, Westergaard T, Helweg-Larsen K et al. Induced abortion and the risk of breast cancer. New England Journal of Medicine 1997; 336(2):81–85.

28. Hartge P. Abortion, breast cancer, and epidemiology. New England Journal of Medicine 1997; 336(2):127–128.

29. Hatch EE, Palmer JR, Titus-Ernstoff L, Noller KL, Kaufman RH, Mittendorf R et al. Cancer risk in women exposed to diethylstilbestrol in utero. Journal of The American Medical Association 1998; 280(7):630–634.

30. Colton T, Greenberg ER, Noller K, Resseguie L, Van Bennekom C, Heeren T et al. Breast cancer in mothers prescribed diethylstilbestrol in pregnancy. Further follow-up. Journal of The American Medical Association 1993; 269(16):2096–2100.

31. Hadjimichael OC, Meigs JW, Falcier FW, Thompson WD, Flannery JT. Cancer risk among women exposed to exogenous estrogens during pregnancy. Journal of the National Cancer Institute 1984; 73(4):831–834.

32. Greenberg ER, Barnes AB, Resseguie L, Barrett JA, Burnside S, Lanza LL et al. Breast cancer in mothers given diethylstilbestrol in pregnancy. New England Journal of Medicine 1984; 311(22):1393–1398.

33. Narod SA, Risch H, Moslehi R, Dorum A, Neuhausen S, Olsson H et al. Oral contraceptives and the risk of hereditary ovarian cancer. Hereditary Ovarian Cancer Clinical Study Group. New England Journal of Medicine 1998; 339(7):424–428.

34. Latikka P, Pukkala E, Vihko V. Relationship between the risk of breast cancer and physical activity. An epidemiological perspective. Sports Medicine 1998; 26(3):133–143.

35. Thune I, Brenn T, Lund E, Gaard M. Physical activity and the risk of breast cancer. New England Journal of Medicine 1997; 336(18):1269–1275.

36. Hunter DJ, Spiegelman D, Adami HO, Beeson L, van den Brandt PA, Folsom AR et al. Cohort studies of fat intake and the risk of breast cancer—a pooled analysis. New England Journal of Medicine 1996; 334(6):356–361.

37. Hunter DJ, Hankinson SE, Laden F, Colditz GA, Manson JE, Willett WC et al. Plasma organochlorine levels and the risk of breast cancer. New England Journal of Medicine 1997; 337(18):1253–1258.

38. Hoyer AP, Grandjean P, Jorgensen T, Brock JW, Hartvig HB. Organochlorine exposure and risk of breast cancer. The Lancet 1998; 352(9143):1816–1820.

39. Morabia A, Bernstein M, Heritier S, Khatchatrian N. Relation of breast cancer with passive and active exposure to tobacco smoke. American Journal of Epidemiology 1996; 143(9):918–928.

40. Lash TL, Aschengrau A. Active and passive cigarette smoking and the occurrence of breast cancer. American Journal of Epidemiology 1999; 149(1):5–12.

41. Bryant H, Brasher P. Breast implants and breast cancer—reanalysis of a linkage study. New England Journal of Medicine 1995; 332(23): 1535–1539.

42. Edelman DA, Grant S, van Os WA. Breast cancer risk among women using silicone gel breast implants. International Journal of Fertility and Menopausal Studies 1995; 40(5):274–280.

43. Bhatia S, Robison LL, Oberlin O, Greenberg M, Bunin G, Fossati-Bellani F et al. Breast cancer and other second neoplasms after childhood Hodgkin's disease. New England Journal of Medicine 1996; 334(12):745–751.

44. Aisenberg AC, Finkelstein DM, Doppke KP, Koerner FC, Boivin JF, Willett CG. High risk of breast carcinoma after irradiation of young women with Hodgkin's disease. Cancer 1997; 79(6):1203–1210.

45. Hancock SL, Tucker MA, Hoppe RT. Factors affecting late mortality from heart disease after treatment of Hodgkin's disease. Journal of the American Medical Association 1993; 270(16):1949–1955.

46. Wolden SL, Lamborn KR, Cleary SF, Tate DJ, Donaldson SS. Second cancers following pediatric Hodgkin's disease. Journal of Clinical Oncology 1998; 16(2):536–544.

47. Hudson MM, Poquette CA, Lee J, Greenwald CA, Shah A, Luo X et al. Increased mortality after successful treatment for Hodgkin's disease. Journal of Clinical Oncology 1998; 16(11):3592–3600.

48. DeVita VTJ. Late sequelae of treatment of Hodgkin's disease. Current Opinion in Oncology 1997; 9(5):428–431.

49. Roberts FD, Newcomb PA, Trentham-Dietz A, Storer BE. Self-reported stress and risk of breast cancer. Cancer 1996; 77(6):1089–1093.

50. Henderson MM. Nutritional aspects of breast cancer. Cancer 1995; 76(10 Suppl):2053–2058.

3. How Cancer Begins, Grows, and Spreads

1. McCarthy KS, Nath M. Breast. In: Sternberg SS, editor. Histology for Pathologists. Philadelphia: Lippincott-Raven, 1997: 71–82.

2. Bishop JM, Weinberg RA. Scientific American Molecular Oncology. New York: Scientific American Medicine, 1996.

3. Lodish H, Baltimore D, Berk A, Zipursky S, Matsudaira P. Molecular Cell Biology. 3 ed. W.H. Freeman & Co., 1995.

4. Mooney DJ, Mikos AG. Growing new organs. Scientific American 1999; 280(4):60–65.

5. Wyllie AH. Apoptosis. Death gets a brake. Nature 1994; 369(6478):272–273.

6. Young S. Life and death in the condemned cell. New Scientist 1992; 25(January):34–37.

7. Ashkenazi A, Dixit VM. Apoptosis control by death and decoy receptors. Current Opinion in Cell Biology 1999; 11(2):255–260.

8. Ashkenazi A, Dixit VM. Death receptors: signaling and modulation. Science 1998; 281(5381):1305–1308.

9. Salomon RN, Diaz-Cano S. Introduction to apoptosis. Diagnostic Molecular Pathology 1995; 4(4):235–238.

10. Wyllie AH. Apoptosis: an overview. British Medical Bulletin 1997; 53(3):451–465.

11. Cotran R, Kumar V, Collins T. Robbins Pathologic Basis of Disease. 6 ed. Philadelphia: W.B. Saunders, 1999.

12. Lindahl T. DNA repair. DNA surveillance defect in cancer cells. Current Biology 1994; 4(3):249–251.

13. Marx J. DNA repair comes into its own. Science 1994; 266(5186):728–730.

14. Ross JS, Fletcher JA. HER-2/neu (c-erbB2) gene and protein in breast cancer. American Journal of Clinical Pathology 1999; 112(1 Suppl 1):S53-S67.

15. Pusztai L, Lewis CE, Lorenzen J, McGee JO. Growth factors: regulation of normal and neoplastic growth. Journal of Pathology 1993; 169(2):191–201.

16. Goldenberg MM. Trastuzumab, a recombinant DNA–derived humanized monoclonal antibody, a novel agent for the treatment of metastatic breast cancer. Clinical therapeutics 1999; 21(2):309–318.

17. Levine AJ. P53, the cellular gatekeeper for growth and division. Cell 1997; 88(3):323–331.

18. Prives C, Hall PA. The p53 pathway. Journal of Pathology 1999; 187(1):112–126.

19. Pillai MR, Kesari AL, Chellam VG, Madhavan J, Nair P, Nair MK. Spontaneous programmed cell death in infiltrating duct carcinoma: Association with p53, BCL-2, hormone receptors and tumor proliferation. Pathology, Research and Practice 1998; 194(8):549–557.

20. Brugarolas J, Jacks T. Double indemnity: P53, BRCA and cancer. P53 mutation partially rescues developmental arrest in BRCA1 and BRCA2 null mice, suggesting a role for familial breast cancer genes in DNA damage repair. Nature Medicine 1997; 3(7):721–722.

21. Kinzler KW, Vogelstein B. Cancer therapy meets p53. New England Journal of Medicine 1994; 331(1):49–50.

22. Marx J. New link found between p53 and DNA repair. Science 1994; 266(5189):1321–1322.

23. Harris CC, Hollstein M. Clinical implications of the p53 tumor-suppressor gene. New England Journal of Medicine 1993; 329:1318–1327.

24. Pietenpol JA, Vogelstein B. Tumour suppressor genes. No room at the p53 inn. Nature 1993; 365(6441):17–18.

25. Evans SC, Lozano G. The Li-Fraumeni syndrome: An inherited susceptibility to cancer. Molecular Medicine Today 1997; 3(9):390–395.

26. Hellman S. Darwin's clinical relevance. Cancer 1997; 79(12): 2275–2281.

27. Adams JM, Cory S. The Bcl-2 protein family: arbiters of cell survival. Science 1998; 281(5381):1322–1326.

28. McDonnell TJ, Beham A, Sarkiss M, Andersen MM, Lo P. Importance of the Bcl-2 family in cell death regulation. Experientia 1996; 52(10–11):1008–1017.

29. Raff M. Cell suicide for beginners. Nature 1998; 396(6707):119–122.

30. Wyllie AH. Apoptosis and carcinogenesis. European Journal of Cell Biology 1997; 73(3):189–197.

31. Jost CA, Marin MC, Kaelin WGJ. P73 is a human p53-related protein that can induce apoptosis. Nature 1997; 389(6647):191–194.

32. Fossel M. Telomerase and the aging cell: implications for human health. Journal of the American Medical Association 1998; 279(21):1732–1735.

33. Campisi J. Aging and cancer: the double-edged sword of replicative senescence. Journal of the American Geriatrics Society 1997; 45(4):482–488.

34. Dimri GP, Lee X, Basile G, Acosta M, Scott G, Roskelley C et al. A biomarker that identifies senescent human cells in culture and in aging skin in vivo. Proceedings of the National Academy of Sciences of the United States of America 1995; 92(20):9363–9367.

35. Axelrod N. Of telomeres and tumors. Nature Medicine 1996; 2(2):158–159.

36. Haber DA. Telomeres, cancer, and immortality. New England Journal of Medicine 1995; 332(14):955–956.

37. Greider CW, Blackburn EH. Telomeres, Telomerase and Cancer. Scientific American 1996; 274(2):92–97.

38. Wynford-Thomas D. Cellular senescence and cancer. Journal of Pathology 1999; 187(1):100–111.

39. Gold JS, Bao L, Ghoussoub RA, Zetter BR, Rimm DL. Localization and quantitation of expression of the cell motility–related protein thymosin beta15 in human breast tissue. Modern Pathology 1997; 10(11):1106–1112.

40. Bao L, Loda M, Janmey PA, Stewart R, Anand-Apte B, Zetter BR. Thymosin beta15: a novel regulator of tumor cell motility upregulated in metastatic prostate cancer. Nature Medicine 1996; 2(12):1322–1328.

41. Albelda SM. Role of integrins and other cell adhesion molecules in tumor progression and metastasis. Laboratory Investigation 1993; 68(1): 4–17.

42. Freemont AJ. Adhesion molecules. Journal of Clinical Pathology: Molecular Pathology 1998; 51(4):175–184.

43. Frenette PS, Wagner DD. Adhesion Molecules—Part I. New England Journal of Medicine 1996; 334(23):1526–1529.

44. Frenette PS, Wagner DD. Adhesion molecules—Part II: Blood vessels and blood cells. New England Journal of Medicine 1996; 335(1):43–45.

45. Shiozaki H, Oka H, Inoue M, Tamura S, Monden M. E-cadherin mediated adhesion system in cancer cells. Cancer 1996; 77(8 Suppl):1605–1613.

46. Barsky SH, Siegal GP, Janotta F, Liotta LA. Loss of basement membrane components by invasive tumours but not by their benign counterparts. Laboratory Investigation 1983; 49(2):140–147.

47. Ziober BL, Lin CS, Kramer RH. Laminin-binding integrins in tumor progression and metastasis. Seminars in Cancer Biology 1996; 7(3):119–128.

48. Garcia M, Platet N, Liaudet E, Laurent V, Derocq D, Brouillet JP et al. Biological and clinical significance of cathepsin D in breast cancer metastasis. Stem Cells 1996; 14(6):642–650.

49. Chambers AF, Matrisian LM. Changing views of the role of matrix metalloproteinases in metastasis. Journal of the National Cancer Institute 1997; 89(17):1260–1270.

50. Andreasen PA, Kjoller L, Christensen L, Duffy MJ. The urokinase-type plasminogen activator system in cancer metastasis: a review. International Journal of Cancer 1997; 72(1):1–22.

51. Demicheli R, Retsky MW, Swartzendruber DE, Bonadonna G. Proposal for a new model of breast cancer metastatic development. Annals of Oncology 1997; 8(11):1075–1080.

52. Swartzendruber DE, Retsky MW, Wardwell RH, Bame PD. An alternative approach for treatment of breast cancer. Breast Cancer Research and Treatment 1994; 32(3):319–325.

53. Sneath RJS, Mangham DC. The normal structure and function of CD44 and its role in neoplasia. Journal of Clinical Pathology: Molecular Pathology 1998; 51(4):191–200.

54. Folkman J. Seminars in Medicine of the Beth Israel Hospital, Boston. Clinical applications of research on angiogenesis. New England Journal of Medicine 1995; 333(26):1757–1763.

55. Folkman J. The molecular basis of cancer. In: Mendelsohn J, Howley PM, Israel MA, Liotta LA, editors. Philadelphia: W.B. Saunders, 1995.

56. Folkman J. Tumor angiogenesis and tissue factor. Nature Medicine 1996; 2(2):167–168.

57. Folkman J. Fighting cancer by attacking its blood supply. Scientific American 1996; 275:116–119.

58. Barinaga M. Designing therapies that target tumor blood vessels. Science 1997; 275(5299):482–484.

59. Freije JM, MacDonald NJ, Steeg PS. Nm23 and tumour metastasis: basic and translational advances. Biochemical Society Symposia 1998; 63:261–71:261–271.

60. Freije JM, MacDonald NJ, Steeg PS. Differential gene expression in tumor metastasis: Nm23. Current Topics in Microbiology and Immunology 1996; 213(Pt. 2):215–232.

4. The Pathology of Breast Cancer: How It Looks Under the Microscope

1. Cotran R, Kumar V, Collins T. Robbins Pathologic Basis of Disease. 6 ed. Philadelphia: W.B. Saunders, 1999.

2. Elston CW, Ellis IO. The Breast. 2 ed. Edinburgh, London, New York: Churchill Livingstone, 1998.

3. Hutter RV. Goodbye to "fibrocystic disease." New England Journal of Medicine 1985; 312(3):179–181.

4. Love SM, Gelman RS, Silen W. Sounding board. Fibrocystic "disease" of the breast—a nondisease? New England Journal of Medicine 1982; 307(16):1010–1014.

5. Moore MM, Hargett CW, III, Hanks JB, Fajardo LL, Harvey JA, Frierson HF, Jr. et al. Association of breast cancer with the finding of atypical ductal hyperplasia at core breast biopsy. Annals of Surgery 1997; 225(6):726–731.

6. Schnitt SJ, Morrow M. Lobular carcinoma in situ: current concepts and controversies. Seminars in Diagnostic Pathology 1999; 16(3):209–223.

7. Page DL, Kidd TE, Jr., Dupont WD, Simpson JF, Rogers LW. Lobular neoplasia of the breast: higher risk for subsequent invasive cancer predicted by more extensive disease. Human Pathology 1991; 22(12):1232–1239.

8. Rosen PP, Kosloff C, Lieberman PH, Adair F, Braun DW, Jr. Lobular carcinoma in situ of the breast. Detailed analysis of 99 patients with average follow-up of 24 years. American Journal of Surgical Pathology 1978; 2(3):225–251.

9. Urban JA. Bilaterality of cancer of the breast. Biopsy of the opposite breast. Cancer 1967; 20(11):1867–1870.

10. Paul Peter Rosen. Rosen's Breast Pathology. Lippincott Williams & Wilkins Publishers, 1996.

11. Paul Peter Rosen. Breast Pathology: Diagnosis by Needle Core Biopsy. Lippincott Williams & Wilkins Publishers, 1999.

12. Fattaneh A. Tavassoli. Pathology of the Breast. Appleton & Lange, 1999.

13. Melvin J. Silverstein (editor). Ductal Carcinoma in Situ of the Breast. Lippincott, Williams & Wilkins, 1999.

5. Mammography and Screening: The Key to Prevention?

1. Giger ML, Pelizzari CA. Advances in tumor imaging. Scientific American 1996; 275(3):110–112.

2. Simonetti G, Cossu E, Montanaro M, Caschili C, Giuliani V. What's new in mammography. European Journal of Radiology 1998; 27 Suppl 2:S234–S241.

3. Karssemeijer N, Hendriks JH. Computer-assisted reading of mammograms. European Radiology 1997; 7(5):743–748.

4. Sox HC. Benefit and harm associated with screening for breast cancer. New England Journal of Medicine 1998; 338(16):1145–1146.

5. Elmore JG, Barton MB, Moceri VM, Polk S, Arena PJ, Fletcher SW. Ten-year risk of false positive screening mammograms and clinical breast examinations. New England Journal of Medicine 1998; 338(16):1089–1096.

6. Rimer BK, Bluman LG. The psychosocial consequences of mammography. Journal of the National Cancer Institute Monographs 1997; (22):131–138.

7. Mammography Quality Standards Act (MQSA). http://www.fda.gov/cdrh/dmqrp/draftcomp.html.

8. Jatoi I. Breast cancer screening. American Journal of Surgery 1999; 177(6):518–524.

9. Maranto G. Should women in their 40s have mammograms? Scientific American 1996; 275:79.

10. Wells J. Mammography and the politics of randomized controlled trials. British Medical Journal 1998; 317(7167):1224–1229.

6. Hereditary Breast Cancer: Looking for Clues in DNA

1. Swift M, Su Y. Link between breast cancer and ATM gene is strong. British Medical Journal 1999; 318(7180):400.

2. Schrager CA, Schneider D, Gruener AC, Tsou HC, Peacocke M. Clinical and pathological features of breast disease in Cowden's syndrome: an underrecognized syndrome with an increased risk of breast cancer. Human Pathology 1998; 29(1):47–53.

3. Akashi M, Koeffler HP. Li-Fraumeni syndrome and the role of the P53 tumor suppressor gene in cancer susceptibility. Clinical Obstetrics and Gynecology 1998; 41(1):172–199.

4. Brugarolas J, Jacks T. Double indemnity: P53, BRCA and cancer. P53 mutation partially rescues developmental arrest in BRCA1 and BRCA2 null mice, suggesting a role for familial breast cancer genes in DNA damage repair. Nature Medicine 1997; 3(7):721–722.

5. Hainaut P, Soussi T, Shomer B, Hollstein M, Greenblatt M, Hovig E et al. Database of p53 gene somatic mutations in human tumors and cell lines: updated compilation and future prospects. Nucleic Acids Research 1997; 25(1):151–157.

6. Prives C, Hall PA. The p53 pathway. Journal of Pathology 1999; 187(1):112–126.

7. Schweitzer S, Hogge JP, Grimes M, Bear HD, de Paredes ES. Cowden disease: a cutaneous marker for increased risk of breast cancer. American Journal of Roentgenology 1999; 172(2):349–351.

8. Marsh DJ, Dahia PL, Caron S, Kum JB, Frayling IM, Tomlinson IP et al. Germline PTEN mutations in Cowden syndrome–like families. Journal of Medical Genetics 1998; 35(11):881–885.

9. Nelen MR, Kremer H, Konings IB, Schoute F, van Essen AJ, Koch R et al. Novel PTEN mutations in patients with Cowden disease: absence of clear genotype-phenotype correlations. European Journal of Human Genetics 1999; 7(3):267–273.

10. Miki Y, Swensen J, Shattuck-Eidens D, Futreal PA, Harshman K, Tavtigian S et al. A strong candidate for the breast and ovarian cancer susceptibility gene BRCA1. Science 1994; 266(5182):66–71.

11. Futreal PA, Liu Q, Shattuck-Eidens D, Cochran C, Harshman K,

Tavtigian S et al. BRCA1 mutations in primary breast and ovarian carcinomas. Science 1994; 266(5182):120–122.

12. Wooster R, Bignell G, Lancaster J, Swift S, Seal S, Mangion J et al. Identification of the breast cancer susceptibility gene BRCA2 [published erratum appears in Nature 1996 Feb 22; 379(6567):749]. Nature 1995; 378(6559):789–792.

13. Wooster R, Neuhausen SL, Mangion J, Quirk Y, Ford D, Collins N et al. Localization of a breast cancer susceptibility gene, BRCA2, to chromosome 13q12-13. Science 1994; 265(5181):2088–2090.

14. Mohammed SN, Smith P, Hodgson SV, Fentiman IS, Miles DW, Barnes DM et al. Family history and survival in premenopausal breast cancer. British Journal of Cancer 1998; 77(12):2252–2256.

15. Marcus JN, Watson P, Page DL, Narod SA, Lenoir GM, Tonin P et al. Hereditary breast cancer: pathobiology, prognosis, and BRCA1 and BRCA2 gene linkage. Cancer 1996; 77(4):697–709.

16. Ansquer Y, Gautier C, Fourquet A, Asselain B, Stoppa-Lyonnet D. Survival in early-onset BRCA1 breast-cancer patients. Institut Curie Breast Cancer Group. The Lancet 1998; 352(9127):541.

17. Verhoog LC, Brekelmans CT, Seynaeve C, van den Bosch LM, Dahmen G, van Geel AN et al. Survival and tumour characteristics of breast-cancer patients with germline mutations of BRCA1. The Lancet 1998; 351(9099):316–321.

18. Schrag D, Kuntz KM, Garber JE, Weeks JC. Decision analysis—effects of prophylactic mastectomy and oophorectomy on life expectancy among women with BRCA1 or BRCA2 mutations [published erratum appears in New England Journal of Medicine 1997 Aug 7; 337(6):434]. New England Journal of Medicine 1997; 336(20):1465–1471.

19. Goldman LD, Goldwyn RM. Some anatomical considerations of subcutaneous mastectomy. Plastic and Reconstructive Surgery 1973; 51(5):501–505.

20. Grann VR, Whang W, Jacobson JS, Heitjan DF, Antman KH, Neugut AI. Benefits and costs of screening Ashkenazi Jewish women for BRCA1 and BRCA2. Journal of Clinical Oncology 1999; 17(2): 494–500.

21. Hartmann LC, Schaid DJ, Woods JE, Crotty TP, Myers JL, Arnold PG et al. Efficacy of bilateral prophylactic mastectomy in women with a family history of breast cancer. New England Journal of Medicine 1999; 340(2):77–84.

22. Eisen A, Weber BL. Prophylactic mastectomy—the price of fear. New England Journal of Medicine 1999; 340(2):137–138.

23. Narod SA, Risch H, Moslehi R, Dorum A, Neuhausen S, Olsson H et al. Oral contraceptives and the risk of hereditary ovarian cancer. Hered-

itary Ovarian Cancer Clinical Study Group. New England Journal of Medicine 1998; 339(7):424–428.

24. Collins FS. BRCA1—lots of mutations, lots of dilemmas. New England Journal of Medicine 1996; 334(3):186–188.

25. Casey G. The BRCA1 and BRCA2 breast cancer genes. Current Opinion in Oncology 1997; 9(1):88–93.

26. Shattuck-Eidens D, Oliphant A, McClure M, McBride C, Gupte J, Rubano T et al. BRCA1 sequence analysis in women at high risk for susceptibility mutations. Risk factor analysis and implications for genetic testing. Journal of the American Medical Association 1997; 278(15):1242–1250.

27. FitzGerald MG, MacDonald DJ, Krainer M, Hoover I, O'Neil E, Unsal H et al. Germ-line BRCA1 mutations in Jewish and non–Jewish women with early-onset breast cancer. New England Journal of Medicine 1996; 334(3):143–149.

28. Struewing JP, Hartge P, Wacholder S, Baker SM, Berlin M, McAdams M et al. The risk of cancer associated with specific mutations of BRCA1 and BRCA2 among Ashkenazi Jews. New England Journal of Medicine 1997; 336(20):1401–1408.

29. Krainer M, Silva-Arrieta S, FitzGerald MG, Shimada A, Ishioka C, Kanamaru R et al. Differential contributions of BRCA1 and BRCA2 to early-onset breast cancer. New England Journal of Medicine 1997; 336(20):1416–1421.

30. American Cancer Society. Internet site for information on breast cancer genes. (2000). http://www2.cancer.org/ bcn/re_genetics.html

31. Wilkie T. Genetics and insurance in Britain: why more than just the Atlantic divides the English–speaking nations. Nature Genetics 1998; 20(2):119–121.

32. Harper PS. Insurance and genetic testing. The Lancet 1993; 341(8839):224–227.

33. Stix G. Is genetic testing premature? Scientific American 1996; 275(3):107.

34. Miller AB. The public health basis of cancer screening: principles and ethical aspects. Cancer Treatment and Research 1996; 86:1–7.

35. Vineis P. Ethical issues in genetic screening for cancer. Annals of Oncology 1997; 8(10):945–949.

36. Goelen G, Rigo A, Bonduelle M, De Greve J. Moral concerns of different types of patients in clinical BRCA1/2 gene mutation testing. Journal of Clinical Oncology 1999; 17(5):1595–1600.

7. Diagnosis: How Doctors Decide What a Breast Lump Is

1. Heisey R, Mahoney L, Watson B. Management of palpable breast

lumps. Consensus guideline for family physicians. Canadian Family Physician 1999; 45:1926–1932.

2. Staren ED, O'Neill TP. Breast ultrasound. Surgical Clinics of North America 1998; 78(2):219–235.

3. Jackson VP, Reynolds HE, Hawes DR. Sonography of the breast. Seminars in Ultrasound, CT and MR 1996; 17(5):460–475.

4. Steinbrunn BS, Zera RT, Rodriguez JL. Mastalgia. Tailoring treatment to type of breast pain. Postgraduate Medicine 1997; 102(5):183–189, 193.

5. Holland PA, Gateley CA. Drug therapy of mastalgia. What are the options? Drugs 1994; 48(5):709–716.

6. Mansel RE. ABC of breast diseases. Breast pain. British Medical Journal 1994; 309(6958):866–868.

7. BeLieu RM. Mastodynia. Obstetrics and Gynecology Clinics of North America 1994; 21(3):461–477.

8. Conry C. Evaluation of a breast complaint: is it cancer? American Family Physician 1994; 49(2):445–456.

9. Maddox PR, Mansel RE. Management of breast pain and nodularity. World Journal of Surgery 1989; 13(6):699–705.

10. Dowle CS. Breast pain: classification, aetiology and management. Australian and New Zealand Journal of Surgery 1987; 57(7):423–428.

11. Leis HPJ. Management of nipple discharge. World Journal of Surgery 1989; 13(6):736–742.

12. Devitt JE. Management of nipple discharge by clinical findings. American Journal of Surgery 1985; 149(6):789–792.

13. Morrison C. The significance of nipple discharge: diagnosis and treatment regimes. Lippincotts Primary Care Practice 1998; 2(2):129–140.

14. Chaudary MA, Millis RR, Lane EB, Miller NA. Paget's disease of the nipple: a ten year review including clinical, pathological, and immunohistochemical findings. Breast Cancer Research and Treatment 1986; 8(2):139–146.

8. Treatment

1. Hortobagyi GN. Treatment of breast cancer. New England Journal of Medicine 1998; 339(14):974–984.

2. Fisher B, Bauer M, Margolese R, Poisson R, Pilch Y, Redmond C et al. Five-year results of a randomized clinical trial comparing total mastectomy and segmental mastectomy with or without radiation in the treatment of breast cancer. New England Journal of Medicine 1985; 312(11):665–673.

3. Fisher B, Redmond C, Poisson R, Margolese R, Wolmark N, Wickerham L et al. Eight-year results of a randomized clinical trial comparing total mastectomy and lumpectomy with or without irradiation in the treatment of breast cancer [published erratum appears in New England Journal of Medicine 1994 May 19; 330(20):1467]. New England Journal of Medicine 1989; 320(13):822–828.

4. Fisher B, Redmond C, Fisher ER, Bauer M, Wolmark N, Wickerham DL et al. Ten-year results of a randomized clinical trial comparing radical mastectomy and total mastectomy with or without radiation. New England Journal of Medicine 1985; 312(11):674–681.

5. Lichter AS, Lippman ME, Danforth DNJ, d'Angelo T, Steinberg SM, deMoss E et al. Mastectomy versus breast-conserving therapy in the treatment of stage I and II carcinoma of the breast: a randomized trial at the National Cancer Institute. Journal of Clinical Oncology 1992; 10(6):976–983.

6. Fortin A, Larochelle M, Laverdiere J, Lavertu S, Tremblay D. Local failure is responsible for the decrease in survival for patients with breast cancer treated with conservative surgery and postoperative radiotherapy. Journal of Clinical Oncology 1999; 17(1):101–109.

7. Page DL, Simpson JF. Ductal carcinoma in situ—the focus for prevention, screening, and breast conservation in breast cancer. New England Journal of Medicine 1999; 340(19):1499–1500.

8. Bellamy CO, McDonald C, Salter DM, Chetty U, Anderson TJ. Noninvasive ductal carcinoma of the breast: the relevance of histologic categorization. Human Pathology 1993; 24:16–23.

9. Berry DL, Theriault RL, Holmes FA, Parisi VM, Booser DJ, Singletary SE et al. Management of breast cancer during pregnancy using a standardized protocol. Journal of Clinical Oncology 1999; 17(3):855–861.

10. Lazovich D, White E, Thomas DB, Moe RE, Taplin S. Change in the use of breast-conserving surgery in western Washington after the 1990 NIH Consensus Development Conference. Archives of Surgery 1997; 132(4):418–423.

11. Lazovich D, Solomon CC, Thomas DB, Moe RE, White E. Breast conservation therapy in the United States following the 1990 National Institutes of Health Consensus Development Conference on the treatment of patients with early stage invasive breast carcinoma. Cancer 1999; 86(4):628–637.

12. Albain KS, Green SR, Lichter AS, Hutchins LF, Wood WC, Henderson IC et al. Influence of patient characteristics, socioeconomic factors, geography, and systemic risk on the use of breast-sparing treatment in women enrolled in adjuvant breast cancer studies: an analysis of two intergroup trials. Journal of Clinical Oncology 1996; 14(11):3009–3017.

13. Lazovich DA, White E, Thomas DB, Moe RE. Underutilization of breast-conserving surgery and radiation therapy among women with stage

I or II breast cancer. Journal of The American Medical Association 1991; 266(24):3433–3438.

14. Gustavsson A, Bendahl PO, Cwikiel M, Eskilsson J, Thapper KL, Pahlm O. No serious late cardiac effects after adjuvant radiotherapy following mastectomy in premenopausal women with early breast cancer. International Journal of Radiation Oncology, Biology, Physics 1999; 43(4):745–754.

15. Nattinger AB, Hoffmann RG, Howell-Pelz A, Goodwin JS. Effect of Nancy Reagan's mastectomy on choice of surgery for breast cancer by U.S. women. Journal of The American Medical Association 1998; 279(10):762–766.

16. Nancy Reagan's choice of mastectomy seems to have influenced many breast cancer patients. Oncology 1998; 12(5):668.

17. Farrow DC, Hunt WC, Samet JM. Geographic variation in the treatment of localized breast cancer. New England Journal of Medicine 1992; 326(17):1097–1101.

18. Ayanian JZ, Guadagnoli E. Variations in breast cancer treatment by patient and provider characteristics. Breast Cancer Research and Treatment 1996; 40(1):65–74.

19. Krag D, Weaver D, Ashikaga T, Moffat F, Klimberg VS, Shriver C et al. The sentinel node in breast cancer—a multicenter validation study. New England Journal of Medicine 1998; 339(14):941–946.

20. McMasters KM, Giuliano AE, Ross MI, Reintgen DS, Hunt KK, Byrd DR et al. Sentinel-lymph-node biopsy for breast cancer—not yet the standard of care. New England Journal of Medicine 1998; 339(14):990–995.

21. Paszat LF, Mackillop WJ, Groome PA, Boyd C, Schulze K, Holowaty E. Mortality from myocardial infarction after adjuvant radiotherapy for breast cancer in the surveillance, epidemiology, and end-results cancer registries. Journal of Clinical Oncology 1998; 16(8):2625–2631.

22. Paszat LF, Mackillop WJ, Groome PA, Schulze K, Holowaty E. Mortality from myocardial infarction following postlumpectomy radiotherapy for breast cancer: a population-based study in Ontario, Canada. International Journal of Radiation Oncology, Biology, Physics 1999; 43(4):755–762.

23. Silverstein MJ. Ductal carcinoma in situ of the breast. British Medical Journal 1998; 317(7160):734–739.

24. Cancernet. http://cancernet.nci.nih.gov/clinpdq/therapy/Radiotherapy.html

25. National Cancer Institute. Cancer Facts. Radiotherapy. http://cancernet.nci.nih.gov/clinpdq/therapy/Radiotherapy.html

26. BCA web site http://www.medsch.wisc.edu/bca/faq/radiation.html

27. Ragaz J, Jackson SM, Le N, Plenderleith IH, Spinelli JJ, Basco VE et al. Adjuvant radiotherapy and chemotherapy in node-positive pre-

menopausal women with breast cancer. New England Journal of Medicine 1997; 337(14):956–962.

28. Overgaard M, Jensen MB, Overgaard J, Hansen PS, Rose C, Andersson M et al. Postoperative radiotherapy in high-risk postmenopausal breast-cancer patients given adjuvant Tamoxifen: Danish Breast Cancer Cooperative Group DBCG 82c randomised trial. The Lancet 1999; 353(9165):1641–1648.

29. Lippman ME. High-dose chemotherapy plus autologous bone marrow transplantation for metastatic breast cancer [editorial]. New England Journal of Medicine 2000; 342(15):1119–1120.

30. Stadtmauer EA, O'Neill A, Goldstein LJ, Crilley PA, Mangan KF, Ingle JN et al. Conventional-dose chemotherapy compared with high-dose chemotherapy plus autologous hematopoietic stem-cell transplantation for metastatic breast cancer. New England Journal of Medicine 2000; 342(15):1069–1076.

31. Ueda K, Yoshida A, Amachi T. Recent progress in P–glycoprotein research. Anti-Cancer Drug Design 1999; 14(2):115–121.

32. Duhem C, Ries F, Dicato M. What does multidrug resistance (MDR) expression mean in the clinic? Oncologist 1996; 1(3):151–158.

33. Robert J. Multidrug resistance in oncology: diagnostic and therapeutic approaches. European Journal of Clinical Investigation 1999; 29(6):536–545.

34. Berry DL, Theriault RL, Holmes FA, Parisi VM, Booser DJ, Singletary SE et al. Management of breast cancer during pregnancy using a standardized protocol. Journal of Clinical Oncology 1999; 17(3):855–861.

35. The Patient Resource Center. Salick Health Care, Inc. (2000). http://www.cancernews.com/articles/cancer&fertility.htm

36. Understanding Chemotherapy. National Cancer Institute. (1999). http://cancernet.nci.nih.gov/peb/chemo_you/

37. Tamoxifen for early breast cancer: an overview of the randomised trials. Early Breast Cancer Trialists' Collaborative Group. The Lancet 1998; 351(9114):1451–1467.

38. Jonas WB. Researching alternative medicine. Nature Medicine 1997; 3(8):824–827.

39. Cassileth BR, Chapman CC. Alternative and complementary cancer therapies. Cancer 1996; 77(6):1026–1034.

40. Aulas JJ. Alternative cancer treatments. Scientific American 1996; 275(3):162–163.

41. Marc S. Micozzi (editor). Fundamentals of Complementary and Alternative Medicine (Complementary and Alternative Medicine). Churchill Livingstone, 1996.

42. Pelton R, Overholser L. Alternatives in Cancer Therapy. New York: Simon and Schuster, 1996.

43. Janssen WF. Cancer quackery—the past in the present. Seminars in Oncology 1979; 6(4):526–536.

44. Jenkins M. Men's Health 12[11], 126. 1997.

45. NCI Cancernet.Internet site. (2000). http://cancernet.nci.nih. gov/treatment/cam.shtml

46. Astin JA. Why patients use alternative medicine: results of a national study. Journal of The American Medical Association 1998 279(19):1548–1553.

47. Burstein HJ, Gelber S, Guadagnoli E, Weeks JC. Use of alternative medicine by women with early-stage breast cancer. New England Journal of Medicine 1999; 340(22):1733–1739.

9. Prognosis: What Are the Chances of Being Cured?

1. Gould SJ. The median isn't the message. http://www.stat.berkeley.-edu/~rice/stat20_98/GouldCancer.html

2. Amichetti M, Caffo O, Richetti A, Zini G, Rigon A, Antonello M et al. Ten-year results of treatment of ductal carcinoma in situ (DCIS) of the breast with conservative surgery and radiotherapy. European Journal of Cancer 1997; 33(10):1559–1565.

3. Silverstein MJ, Barth A, Poller DN, Gierson ED, Colburn WJ, Waisman JR et al. Ten-year results comparing mastectomy to excision and radiation therapy for ductal carcinoma in situ of the breast. European Journal of Cancer 1995; 31A(9):1425–1427.

4. Bellamy CO, McDonald C, Salter DM, Chetty U, Anderson TJ. Noninvasive ductal carcinoma of the breast: the relevance of histologic categorization. Human Pathology 1993; 24:16–23.

5. Silverstein MJ, Lagios MD, Groshen S, Waisman JR, Lewinsky BS, Martino S et al. The influence of margin width on local control of ductal carcinoma in situ of the breast. New England Journal of Medicine 1999; 340(19):1455–1461.

6. Schnitt SJ, Morrow M. Lobular carcinoma in situ: current concepts and controversies. Seminars in Diagnostic Pathology 1999; 16(3):209–223.

7. Hortobagyi GN. Treatment of breast cancer. New England Journal of Medicine 1998; 339(14):974–984.

8. Cady B. Is axillary lymph node dissection necessary in routine management of breast cancer? No. Important Advances in Oncology 1996; 251–265.

9. Krag D, Weaver D, Ashikaga T, Moffat F, Klimberg VS, Shriver C et al. The sentinel node in breast cancer—a multicenter validation study. New England Journal of Medicine 1998; 339(14):941–946.

10. McMasters KM, Giuliano AE, Ross MI, Reintgen DS, Hunt KK,

Byrd DR et al. Sentinel-lymph-node biopsy for breast cancer—not yet the standard of care. New England Journal of Medicine 1998; 339(14):990–995.

11. Liefers GJ, Cleton-Jansen AM, van de Velde CJ, Hermans J, van Krieken JH, Cornelisse CJ, Tollenaar RA. Micrometastases and survival in stage II colorectal cancer. New England Journal of Medicine 1998; 339(4):223–228.

12. Smith BL. Approaches to breast-cancer staging [editorial]. New England Journal of Medicine 2000; 342(8):580–581.

13. Braun S, Pantel K, Muller P, Janni W, Hepp F, Kentenich CR et al. Cytokeratin-positive cells in the bone marrow and survival of patients with stage I, II, or III breast cancer. New England Journal of Medicine 2000; 342(8):525–533.

14. Paszat LF, Mackillop WJ, Groome PA, Schulze K, Holowaty E. Mortality from myocardial infarction following postlumpectomy radiotherapy for breast cancer: a population-based study in Ontario, Canada. International Journal of Radiation Oncology, Biology, Physics 1999; 43(4): 755–762.

15. Bishop JW, Kaufman RH, Taylor DA. Multicenter comparison of manual and automated screening of AutoCyte gynecologic preparations. Acta Cytologica 1999; 43(1):34–38.

16. Birdsong GG. Automated screening of cervical cytology specimens. Human Pathology 1996; 27(5):468–481.

17. Osborne CK. Steroid hormone receptors in breast cancer management. Breast Cancer Research and Treatment 1998; 51(3):227–238.

18. Fisher B, Dignam J, Wolmark N, Wickerham DL, Fisher ER, Mamounas E et al. Tamoxifen in treatment of intraductal breast cancer: National Surgical Adjuvant Breast and Bowel Project B-24 randomised controlled trial. The Lancet 1999; 353(9169):1993–2000.

19. Osborne CK. Tamoxifen in the treatment of breast cancer. New England Journal of Medicine 1998; 339(22):1609–1618.

20. Lamerz R. Role of tumour markers, cytogenetics. Annals of Oncology 1999; 10 Suppl 4:145-9:145–149.

21. Phillips HA. The role of the p53 tumour suppressor gene in human breast cancer. Clinical Oncology (Royal College of Radiologists) 1999; 11(3):148–155.

22. Freije JM, MacDonald NJ, Steeg PS. Nm23 and tumour metastasis: basic and translational advances. Biochemical Society Symposia 1998; 63:261–271.

23. Ozbun MA, Butel JS. Tumor suppressor p53 mutations and breast cancer: a critical analysis. Advances in Cancer Research 1995; 66:71–141.

24. Ross JS, Fletcher JA. HER-2/neu (c-erb-B2) gene and protein in breast cancer. American Journal of Clinical Pathology 1999; 112(1 Suppl 1):S53–S67.

25. Weiner LM. An overview of monoclonal antibody therapy of cancer. Seminars in Oncology 1999; 26(4 Suppl 12):41–50.

26. Goldenberg MM. Trastuzumab, a recombinant DNA–derived humanized monoclonal antibody, a novel agent for the treatment of metastatic breast cancer. Clinical therapeutics 1999; 21(2):309–318.

27. Shak S. Overview of the trastuzumab (Herceptin) anti-HER-2 monoclonal antibody clinical program in HER-2–overexpressing metastatic breast cancer. Herceptin Multinational Investigator Study Group. Seminars in Oncology 1999; 26(4 Suppl 12):71–77.

28. Weidner N, Cady B, Goodson WH, III. Pathologic prognostic factors for patients with breast carcinoma. Which factors are important. Surgical Oncology Clinics of North America 1997; 6(3):415–462.

29. Hutter RV. Goodbye to "fibrocystic disease." New England Journal of Medicine 1985; 312(3):179–181.

30. Ueda K, Yoshida A, Amachi T. Recent progress in P–glycoprotein research. Anti-Cancer Drug Design 1999; 14(2):115–121.

31. Robert J. Multidrug resistance in oncology: diagnostic and therapeutic approaches. European Journal of Clinical Investigation 1999; 29(6):536–545.

11. The Future

1. Fauci AS. The AIDS epidemic—considerations for the 21st century. New England Journal of Medicine 1999; 341(14):1046–1050.

2. Hartmann LC, Schaid DJ, Woods JE, Crotty TP, Myers JL, Arnold PG et al. Efficacy of bilateral prophylactic mastectomy in women with a family history of breast cancer. New England Journal of Medicine 1999; 340(2):77–84.

3. Schrag D, Kuntz KM, Garber JE, Weeks JC. Decision analysis—effects of prophylactic mastectomy and oophorectomy on life expectancy among women with BRCA1 or BRCA2 mutations [published erratum appears in New England Journal of Medicine 1997 Aug 7;337(6):434]. New England Journal of Medicine 1997; 336(20):1465–1471.

4. Gibbs WW. The prevention pill. Scientific American 1998; 278(6):26–27.

5. Osborne CK. Tamoxifen in the treatment of breast cancer. New England Journal of Medicine 1998; 339(22):1609–1618.

6. Buzdar AU, Hortobagyi GN. Recent advances in adjuvant therapy of breast cancer. Seminars in Oncology 1999; 26(4 Suppl 12):21–27.

7. Vogel CL. Hormonal approaches to breast cancer treatment and prevention: an overview. Seminars in Oncology 1996; 23(4 Suppl 9):2–9.

8. Reynolds HE. Advances in breast imaging. Hematology/Oncology Clinics of North America 1999; 13(2):333–348, v.

9. Duffy MJ, Maguire TM, McDermott EW, O'Higgins N. Urokinase plasminogen activator: a prognostic marker in multiple types of cancer. Journal of Surgical Oncology 1999; 71(2):130–135.

10. Chauveau N, Hamzaoui L, Rochaix P, Rigaud B, Voigt JJ, Morucci JP. Ex vivo discrimination between normal and pathological tissues in human breast surgical biopsies using bioimpedance spectroscopy. Annals of New York Academy of Science 1999; 873:42– 50.

11. Trevathan-Ramirez D. Innovations in breast disease diagnosis. Radiologic Technology 1998; 70(2):197-203.

12. Lippman ME. High-dose chemotherapy plus autologous bone marrow transplantation for metastatic breast cancer [editorial]. New England Journal of Medicine 2000; 342(15):1119–1120.

13. Stadtmauer EA, O'Neill A, Goldstein LJ, Crilley PA, Mangan KF, Ingle JN et al. Conventional-dose chemotherapy compared with high-dose chemotherapy plus autologous hematopoietic stem-cell transplantation for metastatic breast cancer. New England Journal of Medicine 2000; 342(15):1069–1076.

14. Pardoll DM. Cancer vaccines. Nature Medicine 1998; 4(5 Suppl):525–531.

15. Old LJ. Immunotherapy for cancer. Scientific American 1996; 275(3):136–143.

16. Weiner LM. An overview of monoclonal antibody therapy of cancer. Seminars in Oncology 1999; 26(4 Suppl 12):41–50.

17. Borden EC, Esserman L, Linder DJ, Campbell MJ, Fulton AM. Biological therapies for breast carcinoma: concepts for improvement in survival. Seminars in Oncology 1999; 26(4 Suppl 12):28–40.

18. Shak S. Overview of the trastuzumab (Herceptin) anti–HER-2 monoclonal antibody clinical program in HER-2–overexpressing metastatic breast cancer. Herceptin Multinational Investigator Study Group. Seminars in Oncology 1999; 26(4 Suppl 12):71–77.

19. Braly P. Preventing cervical cancer. Nature Medicine 1996; 2(7):749–751.

20. Arlinghaus RB. Vaccines against tumor antigens. Advances in Veterinary Science and Comparative Medicine 1989; 33:377–395.

21. Schafer DF, Sorrell MF. Hepatocellular carcinoma. The Lancet 1999; 353(9160):1253–1257.

22. Sallie R, Di Bisceglie AM. Viral hepatitis and hepatocellular carcinoma. Gastroenterology Clinics of North America 1994; 23(3):567–579.

23. Seder RA, Gurunathan S. DNA vaccines—designer vaccines for

the 21st century. New England Journal of Medicine 1999; 341(4):277–278.

24. McDonnell WM, Askari FK. DNA vaccines. New England Journal of Medicine 1996; 334(1):42–45.

25. Early breast cancer trialists' collaborative favourable and unfavourable effects on long-term survival of radiotherapy for early breast cancer: an overview of the randomised trials. The Lancet 2000; 355:1757–1770.

Index

185